Critical Studies in Risk and Uncertainty

Palgrave's *Critical Studies in Risk and Uncertainty* series publishes monographs, edited volumes and Palgrave Pivots that capture and analyse how societies, organisations, groups and individuals experience and confront uncertain futures.

This series will provide a multidisciplinary home to consolidate this dynamic and growing academic field, bringing together and representing the state of the art on various topics within the broader domain of critical studies of risk and uncertainty. Moreover, the series is sensitive to the broader political, structural and socio-cultural conditions in which particular approaches to complexity and uncertainty become legitimated ahead of others.

It provides cutting edge theoretical and empirical, as well as established and emerging methodological contributions, and welcomes projects on risk, trust, hope, intuition, emotions and faith. Explorations into the institutionalisation of approaches to uncertainty within regulatory and other governmental regimes are also of interest.

Claudine Burton-Jeangros

Experiences of Health Risks

Prevention, Power Dynamics and Inequalities

palgrave
macmillan

Claudine Burton-Jeangros
Institute of Sociological Research
University of Geneva
Geneva, Switzerland

This work was supported by Schweizerischer Nationalfonds zur Förderung der Wissenschaftlichen Forschung (10BP12_232469/1).

ISSN 2523-7268 ISSN 2523-7276 (electronic)
Critical Studies in Risk and Uncertainty
ISBN 978-3-031-65376-6 ISBN 978-3-031-65377-3 (eBook)
https://doi.org/10.1007/978-3-031-65377-3

Cover illustration: Zoonar GmbH / Alamy Stock Photo

This Palgrave Macmillan imprint is published by the registered company Springer Nature Switzerland AG.
The registered company address is: Gewerbestrasse 11, 6330 Cham, Switzerland

To Tony

Contents

1

Introduction: Experiences of Health Risks

The idea of risk has gained widespread influence on how we live. Individually and collectively, in official and mundane activities, risk has become a catch-all concept expected to guide actions toward averting unwanted future situations. Probabilities, as a cognitive tool developed by statisticians, are constantly used to anticipate the future. The appeal of these predictions is supported by widespread aspirations for control over adverse events. Nevertheless, if risk started to shape the social fabric of societies several decades ago, its ambition to improve society and people's circumstances keeps being challenged.

If for many, risk is a tool that should generate undisputable consensus over how to act, the assumption that knowing more about risks is necessarily beneficial can be challenged at the light of the societal disputes regularly generated by the anticipation of harm. Indeed, risk is a profoundly normative concept. It is used to regulate social activities, to allocate resources to some anticipated harm while it denies or misses other threats. In this book, I argue that recurrent debates about risk exist because most of the time the notion leaves aside the complexity of social processes surrounding actual experiences of vulnerability and danger in society.

C. Burton-Jeangros, *Experiences of Health Risks*, Critical Studies in Risk and Uncertainty, https://doi.org/10.1007/978-3-031-65377-3_1

Some general features of the idea of risk are important to sketch upfront as they contribute to the tensions taking place around the regulation of adverse events. First, risk is intangible. It is a discourse, or a mental construction, about what is likely to happen. It is a prediction based on regularities observed on past experiences. Once misfortune takes place, it is not considered a risk anymore, but it is framed as an event, a catastrophe, a disease, or death. The pervasiveness of risk, as an abstract entity existing only in terms of predictions, illustrates well the fact that we live in a post-industrial context, in which information or knowledge is central. Reflecting the overall quantification of social life, risk probabilities are expected to play a prominent role in the conduct of human lives. However, multiple filters affect both their formulation and their application to real-life circumstances.

Second, risk is tightly associated with the ambition to control future events, as formulated by Bernstein: "The revolutionary idea that defines the boundary between modern times and the past is the mastery of risk: the notion that the future is more than a whim of the gods and that men and women are not passive before nature" (Bernstein, 1996, p. 1). Predictions based on risk calculations are associated with thresholds, standards, and recommendations to guide individual and collective actions across various scenarios, defined as more or less desirable. The authority of science is used to formulate a single course of action that should be consensually preferred. However, depending on their multiple relations with the situation and their other commitments, people often do not agree on what is best and who should be accountable for danger.

Third, there is a profound contradiction between risk as a tool designed to elaborate decisions enhancing collective security through cost–benefit analyses and the promotion of individual responsibility in the modern context. Predictions help to estimate what is likely to happen across a number of people or places and can thus support governments and institutions in policy-making. Considering that adverse events will occur, risk pooling generates solidarity across a group of people to support those who will incur loss. However, the application of probabilistic risk reasoning at the individual level or for single cases is not operative, regardless of the odds of disease, death, or catastrophe. Individual autonomy and collective risk regulation are thus not easy to combine.

Fourth, risk introduces a disconnection between increased expectations of safety and persistent experiences of harm. Risk has indeed brought many benefits, as assessed by a range of social, economic, and health indicators. However, predictions are constantly challenged by unexpected crises, unforeseen events, or low-probability accidents. From the Chernobyl accident in the 1980s to the recent COVID-19 pandemic, the repetition of crises in multiple forms and domains keeps questioning the promises raised by risk management. This disconnection contributes to discrediting the very idea of risk and the trust that experts and institutions had gained over the first part of the twentieth century.

By asserting that nothing happens by chance, risk profoundly impacts society. However, risk only provides a map, reducing the complexity of the world to a limited number of dimensions. Risk is not the territory, the actual conditions in which people experience illness, suffering, and misfortune. My aim is to discuss this tension.

On the one hand, conventional or formal risk management, supported by the increasing capacity to predict harm for human lives and their environments thanks to risk probabilities, has developed a generic model to control the adverse consequences of anticipated threats based on cost–benefit trade-offs. The characteristics of this model include notably being top-down, intellectual, abstract, rational, and quantitative. It gained legitimacy in organizing human activities in the best collective interest and progressively expanded across all life domains. However, its promises remain constantly challenged by its difficulty in fully anticipating threats—which risks should be measured?—and societal reactions—how will people respond to forecasted danger?

In this book, I propose to focus on 'experiences of health risks' to better understand how people domesticate their personal vulnerability, including material, affective, symbolic, and interpersonal elements. This approach considers that they have to turn the abstract or elusive category of risk into something that they can relate to and therefore may act upon. Indeed, risk brings discontinuity or disorder, questioning aspirations for continuity in social life. Thus, people have to integrate unforeseen danger into their routines, possibly revisiting these or accepting them despite them being labeled dangerous. In addition, they make connections with tangible elements, such as their past experiences, their personal conditions, or current societal concerns to gain some grip over this unsettling idea. Being interested in experiences of risk implies to consider these within their related institutional environments which, beyond information, provide rules and recommendations, possibly sanctions. In addition, these experiences are shaped by constant interactions with others, who in their different social roles—as relatives, friends, or professionals—validate some risk interpretations and actions while they devalue others. These relations can generate both conflicts and alliances among people facing potential harm.

In relation with my own research, I focus my attention on people's experiences with regard to health risks, a domain in which risk expansion has been particularly prolific, from individual genetic risks to global pandemic risks. In recent decades, health has indeed gained much scientific, mediatic, and societal attention. Continuous gains in postponing death triggered interest in the anticipation of disease and the promotion of health. Health, as experienced in individual bodies, is situated at the crossroad of biological, social, and political processes. It thus occupies a number of disciplines analyzing it under their specific lenses. As a sociologist, I am interested in the multiple and multifold social processes taking place around health issues. In the context of the HIV/AIDS epidemic, the stigmatization of infected persons early on was considered a challenge as large as the diffusion of the virus. More recently, the World Health Organization warned that the infodemic surrounding the COVID-19 pandemic was as much a threat as the virus itself. These two examples show how risk probabilities have social consequences.

I aim to show how the social sciences contribute to the understanding of health risk prevention. Following Mol (1998), who considers pathology to be a lived reality, or Kleinman (1978), who asserts that illness is the lived experience of disease, I focus my attention on the lived reality of health risks. In addition to being an abstract prediction, being at risk has concrete implications for people's lives, questioning their confidence in their own bodies and their capacity to fill their social roles. In the health domain, science and medicine play important roles, as their position often prevails over others. Their perspective is pervaded by a narrative dominated by a number of assumptions, including scientific reason as a straightforward precursor to collective solutions, people as maximizers of their own interest in every circumstance, and a specific set of values. However, examining experiences of health risk and uncertainty unveils the situated character of prevention campaigns, their underlying power dynamics, and their relations with health inequalities.

My goal is to understand how people in diverse positions, as members of the general public or professionals, actually think, act, and interact around experiences of risk. Influential scholars, such as Beck (1992), Douglas (1985, 1995), Ewald (1986), and Giddens (1990, 1991), have described the social transformations leading to the emergence of modern risk culture(s). However, their thinking has remained mostly abstract, and here, I wish to connect the social theories of risk propositions with empirical studies focused on health risk experiences. These studies help describe the challenges people encounter when they try to make sense of risk, while taking into account the social influences that affect their reactions.

To better understand how people actually handle health-related risks, I address the following questions in the upcoming chapters. In Chap. 2, how do people make sense of risks through multiple forms of knowledge? In Chap. 3, what is the role of emotions associated with risks? In Chap. 4, how are actions adopted to respond to risks justified? In Chap. 5, how is risk prevention shaped by moral judgments in social interactions? In Chap. 6, how do social structures expose and protect individuals differently? In each chapter, a first part brings together theoretical elements, starting with sociological theory, followed by social theories of risk and sociology of health insights. The second part presents empirical findings to illustrate recurrent challenges across risks and contexts. I mostly discuss health risks in affluent countries, but I sometimes adopt a broader scope such as when addressing re-emerging infectious diseases. Attention is given to studies focused on members of the public but also to the role of professionals in institutions, to emphasize how health prevention takes place amidst relations, characterized by consensus or conflicts depending on the issues tackled.

The COVID-19 pandemic clearly revived societal debates about risk, uncertainty, precaution, mobilization of science, and resistance to experts' views. These recent debates only expanded questions that have already been present for a while. In this book, I follow health risks over time and settings to document contrasting experiences attached to them across society.

References

Beck, U. (1992). *Risk society. Towards a new modernity*. Sage. [1986: first edition in German *Risikogesellschaft*].

Bernstein, P. L. (1996). *Against the gods. The remarkable story of risk*. John Wiley & Sons.

Douglas, M. (1985). *Risk acceptability according to the social sciences*. Routledge & Kegan Paul.

Douglas, M. (1995). Risk and blame. In M. Douglas (Ed.), *Risk and blame. Essays in cultural theory* (pp. 3–21). Routledge.

Ewald, F. (1986). *L'Etat providence*. Bernard Grasset.

Giddens, A. (1990). *The consequences of modernity*. Polity Press.

Giddens, A. (1991). *Modernity and self-identity in the late modern age*. Polity Press.

Kleinman, A. (1978). Concepts and a model for the comparison of medical systems as cultural systems. *Social Science & Medicine. Part B: Medical Anthropology, 12*, 85–93. https://doi.org/10.1016/0160-7987(78)90014-5

Mol, A. (1998). Lived reality and the multiplicity of norms: A critical tribute to George Canguilhem. *Economy and Society, 27*(2–3), 274–284. https://doi.org/10.1080/03085149800000020

2

Knowledge, Uncertainty, and Ignorance Around Health Risks

Introduction

Risk is associated with science as a dominant institution in modern societies. Formal risk knowledge, based on scientific reasoning, is expected to guide human action in a wide range of domains with the intention to avert future harm. The capacity to calculate odds, valued by experts and institutions, is associated with the prevention of risks as a widely shared principle for the organization of individual and collective lives.

Challenging the assumption that the expansion of formal risk knowledge is necessarily beneficial, I describe in this chapter how social contexts matter in the production, circulation, and reception of such knowledge. Risk as an abstract idea raises attention before harm is actually present. At the same time, it highlights the extent and permanence of uncertainty, namely, what is not yet known or even knowable. These features of risk evidence are prone to generate controversies in society. In addition to the increasing awareness of difficulties in estimating probabilities that can help predict future misfortune, making sense of the constantly increasing amount of risk knowledge is challenging. This chapter intends to show how, over the past decades, the proliferation of the idea

C. Burton-Jeangros, *Experiences of Health Risks*, Critical Studies in Risk and Uncertainty, https://doi.org/10.1007/978-3-031-65377-3_2

of risk has contributed to transforming the relationships between science and society in general and to undermining the authority of formal or quantitative knowledge.

Across a range of health risks, including lifestyles, genetic or cancer screening, exposure to environmental threats, and infectious diseases, formal risk knowledge is constantly extending with the development of biomedical and epidemiological research. At the same time, this extension continues to create new concerns. In addition to the difficulties reported by people who have to make decisions based on predicted risks, the logic of risk continues to expand the scope of possible actions. Consequently, it creates opportunities for conflicts across contrasted views about the best ways to promote and protect health. In addition, influences affecting the production and circulation of knowledge, or its manipulation to serve situated interests, suggest that multiple social filters affect how risk knowledge is convened in the elaboration of recommendations to protect individual and public health.

I am interested in how social actors, across their different positions and circumstances, praise, challenge, complement, or manipulate tools offered by probabilistic thinking. Against efforts of science to delimit and establish solid facts on possible threats, thus usually looking at them as isolated problems, social actors constantly navigate across a number of health issues. They are regularly confronted to these at their own personal level or as these issues affect people they know, but also to global threats debated across multiple communication channels. By discussing a number of situations, defined as public health or clinical risks, in their real-life application, I am interested in how the shortcomings of formal health risk knowledge contribute to a questioning of the value of science.

In the first part of the chapter, I present elements of sociology of knowledge and social theories of risk to sketch the background against which the evidence about health-related risks has widely expanded. Then, using empirical illustrations from a range of health domains, I discuss how knowing about risks is generating multiple challenges at both the individual and collective levels.

Risk Knowledge Applied to Health

Sociology of Risk Knowledge

For social scientists, the production of knowledge is not a natural and universal process of accumulation that goes unchallenged. Rather, they are interested in what counts as knowledge, whose claims are considered most relevant, and how knowledge circulates in society. This means that the status of different forms of knowledge varies across contexts, reflecting social hierarchies and shaping expected interactions across social groups (Berger & Luckmann, 1991 [1966]). In this section, I first revisit how probabilistic thinking became so dominant and how its success was approached by social scientists.

The Scientific Approach to Risk

In the process of disenchantment of the world described by Max Weber (1964 [1904]), science—or formal knowledge—took over the role previously played by religion and magic in sense-making. Modern secular societies favor explanations of the environment and human activities based on experimentation, systematic data collection, and analysis. These techniques are expected to produce knowledge that evacuates unexpected and mysterious forces and offers control over events (Weber, 1963 [1919]). Dismissing the value of common-sense knowledge, scientists focus on regularities to formulate abstract generalizations. Over the Enlightenment process leading to a rationalization of natural and social life, science has become an authoritative system of knowledge. This implied formulating claims of a 'universalized truth' valid at the worldwide scale, independent of local circumstances (Swidler & Arditi, 1994). This was made possible by the existence of institutions and people who gained sufficient authority in establishing the truth and in arbitrating disputes. Since science started to define what is actually thinkable, Michel Foucault (1989 [1966]) associated such authority with power. In modern societies characterized by functional specialization and rationality, science turned into expertise summoned to guide the organization of social life. Its dominant position was initially reinforced by the limited circulation of formal knowledge, whose access was restricted through dedicated channels and closed to the general public.

Through systematic observations of the past and the development of statistical tools, science progressively became a dominant institution in the management of the future through risks calculated as probabilities offering quantified measures of the likelihood of specific events (Bernstein, 1996). In risk management, preventive actions are defined as the joint evaluation of the probability of an event and its expected consequences (Aven & Renn, 2009). Cost–benefit analyses define possible interventions as a trade-off between positive and negative consequences of any activity. Turning past unspecified dangers into calculable risks (Castel, 1983) led to major improvements in safety and security in all systems supporting people's lives. The capacity to calculate risks and thus to predict adverse events was crucial in the development of compensation mechanisms through insurance and welfare systems (Ewald, 1986). Over the course of the twentieth century, risk analysis has been increasingly and systematically summoned to govern all human activities, such as public transport systems, nuclear plants, and everyday mundane activities, as well as a tool for the regulation of public institutions. Over the past century, formal risk knowledge has become ubiquitous and self-evident, and the identification of potential threats turned into a key pillar of individual and collective action. It follows an overall taken-for-granted quantification of social life, to which considerable social and intellectual resources are allocated (Espeland & Stevens, 2008).

Following the growing success of a probabilistic view of the world, formal risk management is equated with reason and rationality. Experimental and quantitative research designs purposively reduce the complexity of the world to identify regularities that help to calculate risks and to act preventively on hazards. The dissenting views formulated by members of the public regarding the safety of technology and the impact of human activities on the environment, hence statements questioning science, have been attributed to a lack of rationality or to emotions, both of which are considered antithetical to modern society and to science. Studies on risk perceptions initiated in the 1960s (Slovic, 1992) attributed systematic gaps between experts and members of the public to the latter's cognitive deficits. Considering human activities under the lens of the rational actor model, proper education of the public or risk numeracy was deemed the solution to eliminate this gap and to reach social consensus over risk issues (Leiss, 1996). Risk communication, set up as a component of risk management, was then conceptualized as the last stage occurring after scientific and technical processes, aiming at informing and convincing the general public or specifically concerned groups about relevant actions to reduce risks.

Over the twentieth century, formal risk knowledge driven by faith in progress and science had a massive impact on society's organization and cultural background. Through the elaboration of guidelines, thresholds, recommendations, risk management broadly affected social norms by suggesting adequate ways to think and act toward the future. In addition, the ambitions of risk management fueled a zero risk narrative and a never-ending quest for safety: "in contemporary society, we can never feel safe or healthy enough" (Furedi, 2009, p. 217). Reflexive or post hoc assessments of action in light of available evidence often associate the occurrence of any unwanted event with human failure. While expanding insurance mechanisms provide protection against their negative consequences, each of these events still incarnates a missed opportunity for prevention. It most often leads to evaluations of the accountability of those—individuals in their private lives or officials in their professional positions—who should have averted the adverse outcome.

However, this dominant perspective, considering the future to be manageable and under human control, continues to be challenged by alternative ways to approach danger and uncertainty. Hence, recurrent dilemmas associated with risk management prompted developments in the social theories of risks.

The Social Theory Approaches to Risks

The growing influence of risk has led social scientists to scrutinize its impact on modern societies (Short, 1984). Amidst their diverse contributions, I focus here on elements related to the role of knowledge in risk management.

In his acclaimed book *Risk Society*, Beck (1992) contended that modern societies now have to address the management of the risks created by the developments of technology and science. He framed increasing social preoccupations toward nuclear energy and the environment as the result of manufactured risks, that is, those new dangers generated by the development of technologies in industrial society. With Giddens (1990), he emphasized the globalization of risks, alongside important socioeconomic transformations occurring at the worldwide scale. As illustrated by the Chernobyl accident, such invisible and distant risks could only be grasped through mediated knowledge elaborated by specialists. Since then, widespread awareness of global risks has been sustained by analyses and guidance developed by international agencies, such as the OECD report on systemic emergent risks (OECD, 2003) or the annual report on global risks of the World Economic Forum since 2006 (World Economic Forum, 2023). In parallel, "risk profiling" started to cover increasingly everyday life and intimate spheres, including health aspects (Giddens, 1991), under the assumption that individuals would benefit from any information about the risks they are exposed to.

At the same time, this process of constant expansion of risk knowledge, inherent to scientific efforts, rendered visible the limits of what is known and shed light on what is not known (Beck, 1992). According to the distinction between risk and uncertainty, some events can be predicted based on existing data related to previous circumstances, while others cannot be quantified due to the absence of any past occurrence. This distinction, which was formulated by the economist Knight in the early 1920s, was overshadowed by rapid scientific progress and concomitant developments in risk management. Indeed, in the middle of the twentieth century, sociologists Moore and Tumin wrote, "Ignorance is commonly viewed today as the natural enemy of stability and orderly progress in social life" (Moore & Tumin, 1949, p. 787). Nevertheless, a few decades later, the social theories of risk emphasized the persistence or even extension of nonknowledge as a result of the constant expansion of science. Scholarship on uncertainty and ignorance (Gross & McGoey, 2015; Proctor & Schiebinger, 2008) developed to address the complexity of nonknowledge. In addition to attention given to uncertainty and hence to what is not known or knowable, social studies of science contribute to risk scholarship by showing how knowledge is produced, or not produced in the case of 'undone science', while taking into consideration how it is influenced by social, institutional, and material contexts (Frickel & Vincent, 2007; Fujimura & Holmes, 2019).

On the one hand, nonknowledge refers to the absence of evidence itself: no scientific fact merely exists, as is the case with new dangers such as the HIV or COVID-19 viruses when they first emerged. The time needed to collect and analyze data suggests that knowledge and nonknowledge are not opposites but rather situated on a continuum that includes "partial, inexact, uncertain, provisional and uneven knowledge" (Heimer, 2012, p. 19). Indeed, the ever-increasing capacity to collect more data, to pool data across locations, and to analyze them supports the identification of further risks while simultaneously producing manufactured uncertainty (Beck, 1999). Partial and dynamic knowledge regularly places individuals in front of the obligation to make personal or collective decisions, while they know that their decisions will be revisited later in light of new knowledge. I refer to this as uncertainty.

On the other hand, nonknowledge relates to the lack of command over some facts by some people: evidence exists, but it is not known by all. This understanding emphasizes issues related to the circulation of knowledge at multiple levels. First, the ever-increasing specialization of scientists means that they are knowledgeable in narrower domains (Giddens, 1990) and thus struggle to keep up with existing evidence within and outside of their own domain of expertise. The difficulty of distinguishing between personal and collective ignorance is currently exacerbated by the continuously increasing amount of research produced and its rapid diffusion. Second, ignorance studies (Gross & McGoey, 2015) or agnotology (Proctor & Schiebinger, 2008) are interested in the role played by this form of nonknowledge in debates around risks. Here, nonknowledge is conceived as the result of different 'social arrangements' that can either passively end up in the absence of science or actively be produced when the intention to deceive others is present (Pinto, 2015). I refer to this as ignorance.

These social science developments show the transitory nature of formal risk knowledge and the multiple influences affecting its production and circulation. Considering its limited capacity to offer uncontested and stable ways to think about danger, attention given to risks thus inevitably encompasses political dimensions. Douglas' (1985) developments on the social acceptability of risks highlighted that science is not sufficient to generate social consensus on what ought to be done. She suggested paying attention to institutions rather than danger itself to understand how perceptions of risk are shaped: "Since a focus on one kind of danger directs attention away from others, it follows that the perceptual monitoring will not be random, but will be a function of the kind of organization that is being achieved" (p. 55).

Therefore, modern risks associated with technology developments, from nuclear plants to nanotechnologies or genetically modified organisms, to the environmental impact of human activities or to the globalization threats of infectious diseases have not only exacerbated debates about evidence and uncertainty but also revealed how science and its limitations generate contrasted reactions across society. This prompted new policy developments. Participatory technology assessment, consensus conferences, or different forms of lay participation around situations entailing risks (Bogner, 2015; Callon et al., 2001) acknowledge the need for deliberation to ensure democratic processes around decisions related to risks. The emergence of the precautionary principle, which calls for action before evidence is gained or action under uncertainty (Jonas, 1990), also reflects the growing awareness of the limits of formal risk management processes.

The elements discussed above emphasize a growing awareness in society of the shortcomings and dilemmas related to risk knowledge. In this chapter, I show how, beyond scientific expertise and its circulation, knowing about risk is local and dynamic and informed by contexts and experiences. After sketching these theoretical elements about formal risk knowledge in general, I now turn to the more specific domain of health.

Formal Risk Knowledge Applied to Health

In recent decades, there has been a steady expansion of formal risk knowledge around health issues. Prompted by difficulties in treating diseases, this knowledge supported the development of primary and secondary prevention strategies aimed at the general population or narrower categories of persons exposed to specific health threats. At the same time, awareness about the absence of knowledge or uncertainty similarly increased among both professionals and the general public. In this section, I am interested in the consequences for health experiences of this intensified proximity with risk and uncertainty. My account is shaped by the different topics on which I have conducted research over the years.

The Expanding Scope of Health Risks

Alongside changing morbidity and mortality patterns, risks have been calculated to anticipate the onset of disease. The accumulation of data, improved technical and statistical capacities, and technological innovations that offer new opportunities to measure some biological characteristics, such as mammograms or genetic screening, have, for example, jointly contributed to extending the production of formal risk knowledge in health.

Over the second half of the twentieth century, epidemiological developments offered a new understanding of noncommunicable diseases after they became the major causes of disease and death in modern contexts. Etiological pathways often remain uncertain, and epidemiological analyses have identified risk factors associated with the occurrence of cancer and heart disease as prevailing causes of death in affluent countries. After an initial focus on biological factors, such as increased blood pressure or cholesterol, attention then shifted toward everyday behaviors as predisposing factors for disease (D. Armstrong, 2014). Following the emblematic study of Hill and Doll in the 1950s, which established a correlation between smoking and lung cancer among a cohort of British medical doctors, large-scale studies on samples of the general population highlighted the role of lifestyles, including diet, physical exercise, tobacco and alcohol use, as a determinant of disease (Nathanson, 1996).

These observations, which are now self-evident, were then completely new. The way they were then framed by public health institutions (O'Donnell, 2015) emphasized the idea of individual responsibility for health. They led to health education campaigns aimed at modifying what was then labeled risk behaviors. A number of behavioral change models focused on psychological mechanisms likely to trigger individuals' intentions to alter their everyday life were developed at that time (Ogden, 1995). With the simultaneous expansion of mass media, prevention messages could easily be distributed to the whole population. Henceforth, the importance of everyday social practices for health became commonplace, giving individuals a major responsibility in achieving their own good health (Crawford, 1980).

In parallel, secondary prevention strategies supported by probabilistic information have been developed (N. Armstrong & Eborall, 2012). Such programs target groups of the population who are in good health but are defined as being at risk due to their age or condition. Cancer screening was first established with pap smears generalized in the 1970s, followed by mammography screening for breast cancer and, more recently, prostate and colorectal cancer screening. These techniques of secondary prevention offered the possibility to detect early signs of the disease to interfere with its natural history. Prenatal screening has also expanded in recent decades to detect genetic anomalies early in pregnancy, notably through techniques for screening for an elevated risk of Down syndrome among pregnant women (Hammer & Burton-Jeangros, 2013). A more recent expansion of genetic screening was prompted by the completion of the Human Genome Project in 2003. The combination of molecular profiling technologies and data mining strategies has opened up the field of personalized medicine, aiming at tailoring therapeutic strategies to the profile of each specific individual to overcome the limitations of the 'one-size-fits-all' model used thus far in medicine (Rose, 2013). Such genetic screening is notably used in oncogenetics to adjust treatments and identify genetic risks that could also concern members of the family (Caiata-Zufferey et al., 2014). Access to genetic information is not only gained in the medical context since over-the-counter offers for genetic testing have increased over the past years (Saukko, 2018). These various forms of screening share a similar goal, that is, identifying risks early, before any visible symptom.

In addition to these individual and local circumstances, risk thinking has also been at the center of approaches developed to address (re)emerging infectious diseases. After a brief distancing with infectious diseases in affluent countries (Bourdelais, 2003), HIV/AIDS in the early 1980s was followed by a succession of epidemics, including SARS, H5N1, H1N1, Ebola, MERS, Zika (Bourrier et al., 2019; Washer, 2010), and, recently, COVID-19. In the initial absence of medical responses, that is, treatments and/or immunization, public health authorities focused on non-medical, that is, behavioral, measures expecting the population to endorse safe practices. The context of globalization, with its high mobility of goods and people, was seen as particularly conducive to large epidemics and prompted the development of global health as a new discipline. Following a trend initiated by the HIV/AIDS epidemic, emerging infectious diseases have typically been framed under the lens of risk. However, their unfolding also emphasized the extent of uncertainty in the face of new situations, such as HIV in the 1980s and COVID-19 in 2020, for which past data to estimate risks were at first absent (Aven & Bouder, 2020). Epidemics have triggered efforts in epidemiological modeling to address evolving uncertainty (Rhodes et al., 2020; Rhodes & Lancaster, 2022). The performative character of mathematics is important to stress since hypotheses about the extent and speed of virus diffusion are what make a pandemic exist 'here-and-now' even though knowledge is still missing: "Models are deployed to imagine futures of unprecedented diseases which cannot be known" (Rhodes et al., 2020, p. 2).

The expanding accumulation of data and their systematic analysis, exacerbated by recent developments in big data approaches combining biological data, electronic medical records, geospatial information, personal self-monitoring through mobile applications and social media, has contributed to identifying further areas of vulnerability (Mooney & Pejaver, 2018). Indeed, personal digital tools reinforce the monitoring of health risks in everyday life by encouraging individuals to closely control their personal efforts and achievements against the norms of good health. The 'quantified self' (Lupton, 2016) not only provides tailored advice to individuals but also contributes to the accumulation of data.

In summary, people are currently constantly made aware of multiple threats, whether they are behavioral, physiological, or even genetic, that loom over their personal health. In addition to this individualization of health, global forces associated with new epidemic dangers have raised international concern, as shown by COVID-19 measures, as they potentially expose everyone to future harm. This extension of health risks reflects a core characteristic of modernity, and the calculation of risks continues to expose individuals to both globalizing influences and their own personal dispositions (Giddens, 1991). To bring together commonalities across these different risks, I present in the next section how the social theories of risk and sociology of health have commented on the different features of this expanding health risk landscape.

Challenges Associated with Surveillance of Health Risks

Health sociologists have widely discussed this extension of health risks through the elaboration of different concepts. Risks, as abstract generalizations gained from data collected across a large number of people, gave rise to a new government of population health, as described by Foucault (2004 [1978]). The identification and dissemination of risks became a tool to govern individuals through their own self-discipline (O'Malley, 2016). These processes led to the formulation of policies based on abstract correlations used to regulate individual behaviors and collective actions in light of what are defined as problematic situations (Castel, 1983). Armstrong coined the term 'surveillance medicine' (D. Armstrong, 1995) to describe the shift toward the observation of normal populations that emerged at the beginning of the twentieth century, extending the territory of medicine well outside the hospital by introducing routine observations into individuals' everyday lives. Through this process, risk shifted professional and population attention beyond the territory of disease by making health a constant preoccupation, with 'healthism' turning it into an individual responsibility (Crawford, 1980). This constant surveillance of risks is also considered one of the key processes supporting biomedicalization (Clarke et al., 2003), and health has become a personal goal that has transformed into an ongoing project and commodity.

Risks gained sufficient force to redefine the boundary between health and disease, now considered on a continuum of in-between positions defined by potential threats (Bourrier & Burton-Jeangros, 2014). Being at risk, which is currently a commonly shared position, is often associated over the long run with constant questioning of health and sustained attention to possible signs of entry into disease. Concepts such as 'at-risk health status' (Kenen, 1996), 'patients-in-waiting' (Timmermans & Buchbinder, 2010), or 'proto-illness' (Gillespie, 2015) are created by the use made of statistical distributions by health professionals. These categories refer to intermediate states in which people are in good health but whose biological make-up or behaviors have been flagged as making them at greater risk of becoming sick than the average person. In addition to redefining their identities, this status is associated with tasks, regular encounters with the healthcare system, new technical devices, services, and specialists to monitor at-risk statuses. Sociological analyses conclude that the expansion of risks reinforces the power of expert systems, that is, medicine and science.

As in non-health-related domains, the initial approach of probabilities as both chance and risk is now most often focused on the latter (M. Douglas, 1990): from global health risks to local and genetic ones, attention is focused on identifying what could go wrong. In addition, alongside social acceleration mechanisms, the expansion of risks, based on the accumulation of more data and capacities to link information across places, the constant anticipation of the future fuels a sense of urgency. Specialists tend to consider that the earlier signs can be detected and acted upon, the better the response should be. This is the case not only for epidemic outbreaks, but also for biological markers. This generates some problematic side effects, or what Beck (1992) defined as manufactured risks in relation to global threats, as a result of a lower tolerance to biological events or modifications. To name a few, there is a growing awareness that cancer screening entails harm, such as unnecessary interventions and anxiety, that must be balanced against its benefits. This has been approached in terms of overscreening and overdiagnosis (Chiolero et al., 2015; Welch, 2011). In oncogenetics, testing can generate fortuitous results—or incidental findings—regarding risks other than those that were initially sought, producing debates among specialists about the necessity or relevance of conveying this additional risk knowledge to people being screened (Owens, 2022).

The continuous accumulation of data is also creating volatility in guidelines. The acquisition of additional knowledge can modify recommendations based on new cost–benefit trade-offs. Over that process, standards and thresholds (re)define the border between normal and pathological positions, as observed for conditions such as obesity, hypertension, or diabetes. This leads to the inclusion of larger segments of the population in the category of those who need attention (Nicholls, 2013; Skolbekken, 2008). At the same time, forces going in the opposite direction, toward a reduction of situations defined at risk, are also reported. The Swiss statement of HIV experts in Switzerland, published in 2008, indicated that HIV-infected individuals under regular treatment were not exposing their partner to risk (Vernazza & Bernard, 2016), generating ambivalent reactions at the international level. The authors invoked transparency to justify this publication, at the light of potential incriminations of HIV-infected individuals in the transmission of the virus. In cancer screening, a tendency toward a lower frequency of testing (mammography, pap smear, prostate cancer screening) also reflects new considerations regarding the respective benefits and harms of screening (N. Armstrong, 2019), as well as economic pressures to reduce health costs. In the early phases of the COVID-19 pandemic, the repeated revision of measures advocated by health institutions also revealed the extent of uncertainty and the constant evolution of evidence (Vargas et al., 2023). As a last example of fluctuations in official recommendations, variations in guidelines across national contexts are used by some parents as an argument to justify their hesitancy toward vaccinating their children (Attwell et al., 2022).

These variations over time and places, unsettling for the public and professionals who have to adjust to different standards, render visible the political nature of actions defined on formal risk knowledge. Such instability of what “normal” or “at risk” means (Skolbekken, 2008) implies that both institutions and members of the public are constantly exposed to concrete negotiations about the acceptability of risks (M. Douglas, 1985). After discussing the critics formulated by social scientists toward the expansion of formal risk knowledge and the expectations it raises, I now turn to interpretations and uses of risk knowledge in concrete contexts, when social actors have to actually handle such information.

The Production, Circulation, and Reception of Risk Knowledge

This second section of the chapter reports on empirical studies documenting how risk knowledge is shaped, shared, and received in concrete circumstances. First, I propose a synthesis of challenges generated by the application of risk knowledge to individual situations, such as in messages encouraging the adoption of specific behaviors or in health care interactions. Then, the application of risk knowledge in organizational settings is discussed, revealing how undesirable knowledge is discarded or avoided in diverse ways. Finally, I address the challenges of risk information overload.

Interpretations of Health Risks in Their Social Contexts

In several contexts of primary and secondary prevention, individuals are informed by representatives of medical and public health institutions about being personally at risk of future harm. I address here the following questions: How do people actually reflect on this risk knowledge in concrete situations? Which strategies do they use to make sense of this information? The findings I bring together suggest that they reinterpret risk information within their social contexts, anchoring their decisions to what they can actually observe or relate to.

Probabilities Challenged

Risks are calculated through abstract constructs produced by statistical procedures, purposively detaching conditions from their life contexts. In primary prevention messages, this information remains fairly general, while in interactions between health professionals and individuals discussing secondary prevention screening tests, actual probabilities are often formulated. This is the case for prenatal screening procedures and genetic screening (Burton-Jeangros et al., 2013; Burton-Jeangros et al., submitted). In those cases, probabilities not only have individual implications but can also have consequences for others, such as the child-to-be or biologically related members of the family. In this context, people can hardly discard formal risk knowledge since they are often urged to engage with this information.

One can argue that the focus on formal cognitive competencies reflects the socialization of scientists, who learn to think about problems in an abstract way and are detached from ordinary considerations. Research on risk perceptions has emphasized the overall poor probabilistic competencies of individuals in decision-making, and systematic 'biases' impeding a proper evaluation of risks have been described (Slovic, 2000; Tversky & Kahneman, 1974). It regrets the extent of poor judgments among members of the public. Efforts developed to improve risk numeracy are aligned with the ideal type of a 'homo medicus', which considers that individuals make rational choices to maximize their health based on probabilities (Peretti-Watel & Moatti, 2010). This assumption is, however, challenged by empirical studies, including among experts.

In real-life situations, research continues to show challenges associated with risk numeracy. It is observed that medical doctors' risk numeracy is weak (Wegwarth & Gigerenzer, 2018). Furthermore, this study highlights the misleading role of leaflets produced by the pharmaceutical industry and medical journals, even the most prestigious ones, whose communication tends to exaggerate risks. In the general public, people admit that they struggle to make sense of the abstract construct of risk. Some question the elaboration of formal risk knowledge. For example, a pregnant woman presented with a probability of chromosomal anomaly of her fetus directly challenged its relevance, associating it with gambling: "There must be a basis, there must be something reliable and tangible in those numbers, but I have the impression that it is totally… as if I was playing lottery and was getting three pineapples or one gun, one pineapple and one peach […] I am not at all impressed by numbers, well by those numbers" (Burton-Jeangros et al., 2013, p. 11). Similarly, citizens participating in deliberative forums on oncogenetics phrased their perplexity, as expressed by the following participants: "In fact, I did not understand, for real I find that 87% said like this…", "it means nothing" or "for me, it is purely theoretical" (Burton-Jeangros et al., submitted).

This can justify the frequent use of metaphors that people use to make risks more concrete or to tackle uncertainty. Pregnant women undergoing prenatal screening made references to pupils in a classroom or pieces of a jigsaw (Burton-Jeangros et al., 2013); in forums discussing genetic screening, participants used images of cars speeding on the highway or planes crashing (Burton-Jeangros et al., submitted). Overall, these strategies suggest the need to connect abstract risk figures with concrete situations so that they can gain some actual meaning to which people can relate. At the same time, metaphors may serve to make persisting uncertainty invisible. In other words, discarding or re-interpreting risk probabilities might reflect a form of resistance to a formal definition of a situation that is not directly echoed in people's everyday lives.

In addition, the predictive nature of risks means that preventive measures do not exclude the possibility that the threat under consideration will turn into an adverse event for the person; in other words, it could occur regardless of the calculated probability. This has been described as an 'ecological fallacy' by Heyman (1998) since a probability projected at the individual level still leaves consequences open. Across settings, people discuss this persistent individual uncertainty. A low probability is therefore not reassuring. In our study focused on prenatal screening, a pregnant woman categorized as low risk told us that "at this moment, I do not know, maybe I will have a Down's syndrome child, we do not know, maybe I will be the 1 out of 1,600, it is possible" (Burton-Jeangros et al., 2013, p. 12). What these women expressed was their deep conviction that despite risk statements, their future remained open. A man interviewed in the context of a sexual health consultation expressed it this way: "For me, zero risk does not exist. This is why one needs to be careful, since there is always a person who will be that person, the one who was not lucky" (Debergh, 2022, pp. 257–258). While risk knowledge helps define collective action, it does not eliminate the occurrence of adverse events, including for those at low risk. Some people will still fall on the wrong side of the equation and suffer harm, against odds. When this happens, they can become vocal about their personal harm and thus contribute to questioning the arbitrary nature of thresholds (Doron, 2016).

These empirical elements show that people—patients, members of the general public, and health professionals—interviewed by social scientists struggle with probabilities and question the utility of risk thinking. These findings highlight that in real-life situations, cognitive processes based on a rational weighing of costs and benefits are insufficient. To make sense of probabilities, people frequently mobilize past observations and experiences to relate risks to concrete circumstances. Hope, faith, and magic have been described as additional tools to tackle the difficulties of abstract risk knowledge (Brown, 2021; Zinn & Schulz, 2024). Through this variety of references, people are connecting health-related risk decisions to social life and add flesh to a narrow cognitive framing.

Experiential Risk Knowledge

These difficulties in grasping the very idea of risk relate to the fact that it is only a mental image: it 'exists' because abstract knowledge about it has been produced, but it is not a concrete entity that can actually be seen or felt. Thus, people experience a gap between being at risk and their bodily experience of health and disease. Research presented below suggests that they strive to fill this gap by summoning knowledge based on their own experiences and on that shared with others. Indeed, people get to know about the world and events through actual experiences accumulated in everyday life. Observations and recurrences help individuals to conduct their life in an unproblematic manner (Schuetz, 1953). The idea of common sense refers to the knowledge ordinary people use in their everyday life actions. Introduced in the 1950s by social phenomenology, it has gained increasing attention since the 1980s (Swidler & Arditi, 1994).

This common sense or experiential knowledge does not meet the criteria defined for elaborating formal ways of knowing; therefore, it has long been discredited under the pressure of authoritative scientific knowledge. Due to the prestige of medicine, health-related social science research has initially adopted such a position, with anthropologists documenting the 'biased' views of people in distant parts of the world and sociologists reporting on the gap between proper scientific formal knowledge on diseases and 'irrational' perceptions among the public. Moving away from this once dominant view, studies have progressively researched people's own understanding of their health and illnesses, acknowledging the importance of experience (Bjørn Hofmann, 2016; Bury, 1997). Around risks, experiential, embodied, or local knowledge has gained in visibility and status across different domains. Indeed, the illustrations below show how the thinking associated with health, illness, and risk is anchored in the social fabric through actual observations of what can be seen, touched, and shared with others.

In the context of prenatal risk surveillance, some women refer to their embodied knowledge of pregnancy to assess the development of the baby and the potential presence of risks (Browner & Press, 1996; Burton-Jeangros et al., 2013; Markens et al., 2010). Embodied knowledge relates to different phenomenological indicators (e.g., bodily transformations) and often integrates past experience, such as previous pregnancies. In another context, some people informed of their elevated risk regarding blood sugar screening questioned the existence of such an invisible risk and preferred to value their bodily perceptions (Norddal et al., 2022).

In addition, feelings and intuitions are explicitly mobilized to interpret a situation defined in terms of risk. This pregnant woman trusted how she felt about the pregnancy more than the probabilities formulated by her gynecologist. She emphasized her intimate convictions that the baby was fine: "In fact no, I was not worried at all, I was not at all preoccupied… well I told myself that… if there was a problem, I don't know, I would have felt it" (Burton-Jeangros et al., 2013, p. 11). Such references are not only a prerogative of patients but are also encouraged by doctors to their patients who have to make difficult decisions, for example, if they are undergoing amniocentesis, which presents additional risks. In different interviews, doctors praised their patients' common sense and instinct: "people have a good sense, and I believe that one can also trust them a little", or "I believe a lot in people's instinct" (Burton-Jeangros et al., 2013, p. 9). This was again reported in a study on women's decisions related to genetic modifications showing an elevated breast cancer risk: one participant who was counting on her doctor's help to balance complex information reported that "He said that I had to follow my deepest feelings, my instinct" (Caiata-Zufferey et al., 2014, p. 4). These empirical elements confirm that risk thinking is similarly challenging for health professionals who have to support patients' decisions. For them, evidence-based medicine, which aims at standardizing medical practices, implies a shift away from their own experience. However, relying on the 'strength of averages' is challenging in clinical practice (Doron, 2016). Thus, 'gut feelings' (Gigerenzer, 2008) or intuition fills some practical function; anchored in social experiences, they facilitate making up one's mind about complex decisions, such as those expected in the presence of risks.

This importance of sensory experience has been reported for other risks, especially those not quantified by science. In the aftermath of the mad cow crisis and then rising preoccupation with food risks, people elaborated their own rules in everyday life to delineate safe and unsafe food, such as through the selection of food providers (Burton-Jeangros, 2004). Aesthetic elements and references to the taste, appearance, and smell of food were mobilized to categorize what could be eaten or not eaten (Green et al., 2003). In the domain of environmental risks, local communities consider that bad odors, chemical residues observed on the ground after rain, etc., offer better evidence of pollution than does abstract scientific knowledge, which tends to eliminate such risks (Brown, 1987). The literature on air pollution also reports on different forms of sensory awareness, including olfactory evidence and physiological effects (Bickerstaff, 2004). The visible presence of a power plant and the first-hand experience of disease or illness were considered signs of 'tangible evidence', defined as "a specific form of lay knowledge that includes experience of disease and sensory perceptions of exposure" (Scammell et al., 2010, p. 151). Overall, people elaborate meanings that help them overcome the difficulties associated with uncertainty.

Finally, counterevidence, that is, observations of real-life situations going against risk predictions, further weakens the relevance of risk. Such experiences are regularly recollected as proof that the future is indeed difficult to predict. Pregnant women talked about occurrences of fetal malformations in contradiction with prenatal screening predictions. Some challenged the strict norms of alcohol abstinence, while in previous generations, pregnant women who drank alcohol without limitations (including their own mothers) had not delivered children with birth defects (Burton-Jeangros, 2011). Similar justifications have also been mentioned in research dedicated to smoking (Wigginton & Lafrance, 2014). Such observations, based on individual and collective memory, contradict the predictions formulated by probabilities.

These illustrations across risks and places emphasize the importance of local and embodied knowledge and the necessary appreciation of risks by those who are directly exposed. The status of experiential or local knowledge has progressively changed in recent decades. Given the visibility of alternative evaluations of risks, broader attention was given to the community activism of those living in sites exposed to toxic waste. In what was named 'popular or lay epidemiology', people's experience emphasized anomalies, particular cases, and possible susceptibilities that distant experts could not be aware of (Brown, 1992; Wynne, 1996). The value of experience has also been acknowledged regarding the mobilization of activists who played a significant role in shaping experiments in AIDS drug clinical trials (Epstein, 1998). Currently, communication technologies provide unprecedented opportunities for distant people to share their experiential knowledge online. Online exchanges with other concerned people provide immediate answers, and possibly reassurance, while obtaining professional advice would take much longer time (Jurich, 2021). Through regular exchanges about their personal experiences and frequent dissatisfaction in encounters with health professionals, these groups can in some circumstances turn into 'epistemic communities', sharing some local and situated knowledge while calling for the integration of their expertise in policy-making (Akrich, 2010) or in the context of evidence-based activism (Rabeharisoa et al., 2014).

A growing legitimacy of these alternative forms of knowledge can be observed across health risk issues. Initial references to lay knowledge (Popay & Williams, 1996) and lay expertise (Prior, 2003) have been followed by 'experiential knowledge' to reduce the negative connotation associated with the notion of 'lay' (Caron-Flinterman et al., 2005). From paternalistic and asymmetric relations described by Parsons in the 1950s, in which the voices of patients were excluded, members of the public have thus gained increasing credibility (Halloy et al., 2022). Such recognition of experiential knowledge and of lay people's expertise can be seen as the result of the social science research conducted in recent decades. In particular, qualitative studies gave a voice to people's concerns and encouraged the interactive or coproduction of knowledge on risks. As I show in the next section, situations framed in terms of uncertainty, rather than risk, have further contributed to making participatory formats popular.

Evidence, Uncertainty, and Ignorance

After describing people's efforts to make sense of risks potentially impacting their own health, I now adopt a different angle by focusing on the challenges associated with the production of evidence on risk and its circulation across concerned publics. Studies shifting attention to the shortcomings of risk knowledge in institutional or corporate settings address another facet of the experience of risks in modern societies. Ignorance studies or agnotology (Gross & McGoey, 2015; Proctor & Schiebinger, 2008) notably emphasize the deliberate manipulation of knowledge to protect the commercial interests of actors in the private sector, including the pharmaceutical and tobacco industries. In addition, I report on research documenting how passive ignorance in the organizational context allows one to avoid uncomfortable knowledge that challenges prevalent frames.

Organizational Avoidance of Risk Knowledge

Endorsing risk knowledge is not only difficult for individuals informed of their personal risk for developing some disease. It is also a challenge within organizational contexts for those who have to accept a new definition of their reality or environment. Different case studies illustrate how organizations manipulate risk information as a result of omissions or interpretations serving alternative needs. Such an analysis was proposed by Vassy et al. (2007) to understand why institutions failed to avert the consequences of the heat wave in France in 2003, when risks were actually known. They claimed that while heat wave risks had been previously documented, different factors related to the circulation of knowledge contributed to the crisis. First, despite calls for action by a few whistleblowers, health authorities initially underestimated the issue since the situation was not in line with the then prevailing cognitive framing of health surveillance. In the early 2000s, attention was indeed focused on infectious disease risks, which were emphasized in the context of reemerging infectious diseases and bioterrorist threats, while environmental threats were still rarely considered. Therefore, despite the available evidence, heat wave danger was not prioritized over other concerns considered more important at that time. In addition, mistrust toward early data and across professional groups contributed to downplaying the importance of the issue. Finally, the evidence remained scattered, a process exacerbated by divisions across professional and administrative entities.

Twenty years later, when COVID-19 emerged, similar shortcomings were observed. Since the early 2000s, massive resources have been invested in global health institutions and international and national capacities in pandemic preparedness, and many experts were convinced that a pandemic would occur (Lakoff, 2017). However, in early 2020, most countries delayed their initial responses, particularly the United States despite being ranked first on the Global Health Security Index (Lakoff, 2022). Indeed, the management of the global pandemic has fueled important debates about risk, uncertainty, prevention, and precaution (Aven & Bouder, 2020). It became increasingly clear that epidemiological evidence and forecasts about the diffusion of the virus were insufficient to govern collective and individual actions.

Another case study described how, in the context of occupational pesticide exposure in France, a danger previously downplayed, emerging risk knowledge was discarded in institutional settings (Dedieu & Jouzel, 2015). As uncertainty long prevailed in that domain, new evidence documenting the impact of pesticide exposure on workers was domesticated or reinterpreted to fit within the existing institutional context. This study shows how collaboration across disciplines was weakened and research conclusions were dismissed. The capacity of actors working within these organizations to ignore some existing knowledge since it did not fit within their institutional structures was again underlined. In addition, the authors stressed that discarding new risk knowledge resulted in alleviating the administrative structure's responsibility for adverse events, thus avoiding the issue of accountability.

These examples suggest that fluctuating risk knowledge questions professionals in their daily routines. Hence, they sometimes make a selective use of this knowledge. In addition, their organizational contexts, more or less explicitly, contribute to generating some ignorance through the division of labor, rules, and tools, in other words, as a result of bureaucracy.

These findings confirm the difficulty of managing complex accumulating information, both at the individual and collective levels, necessarily leading to mechanisms of simplification. The need of individuals, groups, and institutions to elaborate self-consistent versions of their reality can justify in their eyes their partial use of existing knowledge (Rayner, 2012). Therefore, case studies suggest that not only individuals in their everyday life but also those in position to decide for others manipulate, more or less consciously, knowledge and produce ignorance in relation to risk decisions: "the social construction of ignorance is not only inevitable, but actually necessary for organizations, even entire societies to function at all" (p. 122).

More broadly, these illustrations reveal how the social reception of risk knowledge is organized to make it compatible with people's preexisting environments. Such capacity is indeed at the core of social life, through its permanent work toward maintaining some sense of safety and continuity: "one of the crucial jobs of culture, let's say, is to help people camouflage the actual risks of the world around them – to edit reality so that it seems manageable, so that the perils pressing in on all sides are screened out of our line of vision as we pursue our everyday rounds" (Erikson, 1990, p. 123). In contrast, risk knowledge typically challenges preexisting routines and interpretations of the world. It questions the taken-for-granted normality that individuals but also organizations struggle to put in place. In this section, I showed how the complexity of organizational arrangements, competing interests, unstable and partial knowledge concur to question the relevance of probabilities within organizations.

Deliberate Ignorance as a Result of Commercial Interests

A number of studies have also documented how political and economic influences affect the production of formal risk knowledge itself. I consider that they reveal conflicting interests related to the protection of population health and the importance of power hierarchies in society.

Deliberate production of ignorance has indeed been described by research documenting how corporate organizations have made sure that the risks of their products would continue being considered as low.

Tobacco industry strategies have in particular been scrutinized to highlight how their manifold maneuvers have concealed the danger of smoking and passive smoking. These strategies included an emphasis on scientific uncertainty, support for research favorable to smoking, the recruitment of acknowledged scientists, the creation of echo chamber effects, and attacks on unfavorable scientific research (Fernandez Pinto, 2017). 'Industrial epidemics' of commodities detrimental to health, including tobacco, alcohol, and ultra-processed food and drinks (Moodie et al., 2013), have been observed at the global scale and are associated with the increasing burden of noncommunicable diseases in low- and middle-income countries. A number of strategies acting against public health interests and minimizing health risks have been put in place by the large transnational companies behind such commodities, whose extension has been facilitated by deregulation and globalization. They include influencing research findings, co-opting professionals and policy-makers, lobbying to oppose regulation, and calling for voters' freedom over nanny states (Sacks et al., 2018).

These illustrations show that the gray zone between risk and uncertainty leaves room for the manipulation of knowledge through the active role played by various stakeholders. Across domains, these studies illustrate how the production and reception of science can be manipulated and how policies aimed at protecting populations' health are shaped by contradictory forces. Given the increasing commercialization of academic research (Fernandez Pinto, 2017), these issues bring to the forefront conflicts of interests, to which scientists are not immune. Such maneuvers, unveiled by social science research, contribute to undermining the credibility of science as a neutral and rational way to approach risks. In addition, as they are also brought to light by the media, they shape the cultural background in which health risks are widely discussed.

The Circulation of Risk Knowledge: From Risk Communication to Infodemic

Over the first half of the twentieth century, experts controlled the dissemination of scientific evidence in a context of limited information channels. In its early days, risk communication was also a top-down process of experts informing the public when considered necessary. The massive rise of media outlets and communication technologies over the following decades has fully overturned this one-way communication. Against these important transformations, I discuss how today traditional and social media offer not only major opportunities for the circulation of formal risk knowledge, but also act as a source of criticism and conflictual claims, by providing a platform for competing forms of knowledge.

Risk Communication Challenges

Emerging in the 1980s, risk communication was first modeled as a one-way and top-down process with experts giving advice to the public while acknowledging the importance of integrating the whole society into the risk management process (Renn, 2008). It then rested on the assumption that public opinion could be controlled and would align with expert views if properly designed messages were delivered. However, recurrent controversies about risks, fueled by traditional media and later by social media, have led to rethinking risk communication, now defined as an interactive or two-way process based on information exchange between concerned stakeholders (Höppner et al., 2012).

The tight connections between risk communication and public health (Glik, 2007) have been emphasized in times of health crises, notably global epidemics (Burton-Jeangros, 2019). Guidelines produced by public agencies, such as the Centers for Disease Control and Prevention (CDC) in the United States and the World Health Organization (WHO), emphasize the crucial and multifaceted role of communication, or sharing knowledge, around health risks. The revision of the International Health Regulations (IHR) adopted in 2005 stressed communication as one of the eight core public health response capacities required for IHR implementation globally, implying that capacity in risk communication should be built in each WHO member state.

Indeed, public health crises—for example, epidemics, environmental exposures, food safety, and drug side effects—exist and develop through the circulation of information about risks across society. Media channels act as a resource for public health institutions to disseminate recommendations to the public, especially in the context of crises such as the H1N1 and COVID-19 pandemics. Risks related to distant accidents (e.g., Fukushima) or outbreaks (e.g., Ebola) are being rapidly and massively reported, generating global awareness. Local and global threats are thus constantly brought to the attention of the public, the media making risks exist and people aware of threats, whether they are directly exposed to them or not. Indeed, risks are mostly mediated, by science and by the media (Roslyng & Eskjær, 2017), rather than being personally experienced. Nevertheless, people's attention and emotions are continuously triggered.

In the context of H1N1 and Ebola, interviews with public health officials emphasized their difficulties in responding to the demands of 24/7 media channels over long periods of time (Burton-Jeangros, 2019). Coordination of communication within and across organizations also proved challenging, suggesting that institutions underestimated the resources and competencies needed to meet the expectations of their own guidelines in terms of risk communication. In addition, the norm of transparency often contradicts experts' perception that they are expected to know and who therefore feel diminished when acknowledging uncertainty and the limits of scientific knowledge. As made visible during the COVID-19 pandemic, journalists have continued to prompt scientists to report on science that had not yet been done. In the context of massive scientific research production and social expectations to access evidence rapidly, journalists even started to report on findings before these were peer-reviewed, adding to the cacophony of information circulating about COVID-19 risks.

Indeed, as acknowledged in the risk communication developed by public health agencies, the media have become an essential component of outbreak management, with journalists playing an important role in the diffusion of official information and recommendations (Burton-Jeangros, 2019). However, since the early days of risk management, experts have questioned media reporting on risks, regretting the autonomy of journalists. Indeed, the media do not simply accelerate the circulation of formal knowledge; rather, they also actively report on ongoing controversies, such as vaccine hesitancy, rendering visible alternative evaluations of risks. Journalists' commitment to balancing viewpoints leads them to look for contrasting opinions, which they are likely to find among experts but also among other stakeholders, including members of the public. It has been documented how the tobacco industry, taking this commitment seriously, made sure that diverging views about the risks associated with smoking were carried over to the public, fueling questions about the solidity of scientific evidence (Fernandez Pinto, 2017). In the same vein, it has been claimed that food company marketing displayed in media channels, with its emphasis on consumers' choices, impacts not only consumers but also policy-makers (Henderson & Hilton, 2018).

The role of mass communication media is thus multifold: on the one hand, they are a major player in the circulation of formal risk knowledge in society; on the other hand, they contribute to questioning the value of scientific knowledge in complex issues. I now turn to research suggesting that such ambivalence has been exacerbated by the rise of social media, which offer sources of data contributing to the production of knowledge on the one hand, and opportunities for the dissemination of alternative knowledge on the other hand.

The Media as a Resource for Risk Knowledge Production

In the mid-nineteenth century, industrializing nations acknowledged the value of epidemic surveillance and thus made efforts to standardize reporting procedures across borders (Stern & Markel, 2004). In the context of globalization, the importance of knowing early about emerging infections accelerated the revision of the International Health Regulation at the beginning of the twenty-first century. Indeed, it appears that national governments are, more or less deliberately, slow to report outbreaks, while news networks and the Internet disseminate information at a much faster speed and at the global scale. This potential was identified after an incident in 1994, when the World Health Organization first heard about a plague outbreak in Surat, India, on CNN (Weir & Mykhalovskiy, 2007).

In recent decades, the power of media and communication technologies to gather data on health hazards has challenged previous official and bureaucratic channels. As an illustration, Internet communication helped to identify the SARS epidemic in Guangdong Province in late 2002, an outbreak first concealed by the Chinese authorities (Heymann, 2006). Public health intelligence has thus started to rely on electronic information to identify health events at the global scale to maximize the timeliness of responses to emerging threats (French & Mykhalovskiy, 2013). Next to the revision of the International Health Regulations, different networks (the Global Public Health Intelligence Network (GPHIN) or Global Outbreak Alert and Response Network (GOARN)) emerged to monitor the worldwide web to detect any emerging health crises, including deliberate or accidental release of pathogens and chemical and radionuclear materials. These developments supported a departure from formal risk management toward acknowledging uncertainty and "a preoccupation, in public health discourse, with health events of incalculable pandemic potential" (French & Mykhalovskiy, 2013, p. 181).

Infodemiology, a term combining information and epidemiology, suggests a correlation between electronic communication patterns and population health (Eysenbach, 2009). Its potential for public health surveillance combines analyses of available information on the Internet (offer) and of demands formulated by the public in navigation tools, which reflect emerging issues in specific locations. In addition, ordinary Internet users can actively engage in the collection of data in the context of citizen science projects. As an illustration, the BBC Pandemic project recruited 36,000 volunteers to assess population contacts in spring 2020 (Klepac et al., 2020). This material provided detailed information on contacts by age group in different contexts (home, work, education settings) and characteristics (conversation or physical contacts) important for estimating the COVID-19 pandemic diffusion. In the same vein, apps for digital health, beyond their personal use, offer further opportunities to gather large amounts of data (Mooney & Pejaver, 2018) that contribute to the elaboration of further risk knowledge. At the same time, public preoccupations about the privacy of collected data limit the diffusion of these surveillance tools, as was particularly observed in the case of COVID-19 contact tracing efforts, challenged by public mistrust toward the government intentions (Akinbi et al., 2021).

These various developments reflect the sense of urgency generated by formal risk management. In addition, challenges associated with the capacity of institutions to adequately and timely analyze the large amounts of continuously collected data need to be assessed, particularly so in the era of artificial intelligence.

Social Media as an Enhancer of Infodemic

Today, the Internet offers a knowledge base amplified by open science principles and an interactive space where anyone can share her or his experience and views, making them public after having long been hidden in the private sphere (Conrad et al., 2016). I describe here how, beyond their potential for research with access to large sets of data, digital supports trigger social mobilization.

Connections among concerned people, independently of experts, generate concerns in health institutions since these people might convey information that does not meet scientific standards. The democratization of information production and sharing through the Internet has indeed rapidly been considered a threat by the World Health Organization: since the early days of the COVID-19 pandemic, the organization warned against the overabundance of information. It thus developed strategies to fight infodemic, combining 'true and false' information (Pulido et al., 2020), and its website rapidly offered resources to bust myths and debunk false information. Infodemic has been labeled as a risk in itself, interacting with virus diffusion risks (Krause et al., 2020).

Risk communication challenges have already been investigated in the context of previous epidemic outbreaks, notably the H1N1 pandemic and Ebola outbreaks. Institutions recommended early and intensive communication to counter rumors. However, in competition with multiple sources of information, official agencies strived to saturate communication channels with proper information, but thus contributed themselves to the infodemic (Burton-Jeangros, 2019). On a more positive note, it led some public health agencies to invest more resources in communication and in training their staff to acquire skills and competencies in a rapidly changing landscape of communication technologies.

In parallel, research has developed on misinformation or fake news, which directly questions the authority of science. Misinformation refers to information that is inadvertently false and shared with no intention to cause harm, while disinformation is created and shared with the explicit purpose of causing harm (Wang et al., 2019). Since it is difficult to draw a clear distinction between intentional and unintentional purposes, scholars tend to prefer the term misinformation to the latter as well as to 'fake news', which holds a politicized connotation. This systematic review, conducted before the onset of the COVID-19 pandemic, concluded that on the Internet, the volume of misinformation exceeds the amount of accurate information (Wang et al., 2019). In addition, it showed that health-related misinformation was frequently associated with infectious diseases, including vaccine issues. These preexisting features and controversies are likely to have contributed to COVID-19 infodemic.

Fact-checking aims at verifying claims in the news and on social media (Krause et al., 2020); however, this strategy was hampered in the context of COVID-19 by uncertainty and dynamic knowledge. Communication patterns developed during the pandemic reflected the complex role of traditional and social media in public health crisis management, acknowledging them as important players in the unfolding of re-emerging infectious diseases (Nerlich & Koteyko, 2012). Multiple and contradictory voices coexisted, including those disseminating conspiracy theories on the pandemic. However, defined as "explanations of significant events as secret plots concocted by powerful and malevolent institutions, groups, and/or people" (Earnshaw et al., 2020, p. 1/7), such theories are not new. Multiple similar crises have been documented in the past, with alternative explanations being disseminated in different formats, such as films, books, and music. What is new, however, is that social media not only accelerate the dissemination of conspiracy beliefs but also reinforce the polarization of online communities (K. M. Douglas et al., 2019).

Risk communication guidelines advocate interactive communication between official agencies and concerned communities; however, interactions tend to remain limited (Burton-Jeangros, 2019). In contrast, it has been observed that anti-vaccination sites are more interactive than official websites and thus offer people a chance to raise and discuss their concerns (K. M. Douglas et al., 2019). Alternatively, they support their reflexive monitoring of the multiple types of information circulating in parallel. It has therefore been suggested that in times of crisis and anxiety, conspiracy-related groups might bring a sense of community particularly appreciated by their members (Earnshaw et al., 2020; Franks et al., 2017).

I discussed here how the acceleration of risk information circulation reflects a variety of objectives and serves the needs of different groups in society. I underlined that the media not only disseminate official information, but also respond to multiple concerns raised in competing interpretations of risk and uncertainty.

Conclusion

I discussed in this chapter the controversies and debates surrounding the production, circulation, and reception of formal knowledge elaborated around health risks, shedding light on the extent to which social influences shape the cognitive framing of health risks.

Formal risk knowledge formulates numerical assessments with the goal of improving health: "Targets, rankings, projections, predictions, metrics and audits all establish standards and benchmarks, which serve as coordination mechanisms to stabilize health and populations in particular ways" (Rhodes & Lancaster, 2021, p. 2). It is important to emphasize that the application of risk probabilities and formal risk management has indeed generated important gains in many societal domains. However, ordinary safety tends to be taken for granted in society and in social science research and is often overlooked by the focus on extraordinary or poorly managed risks (Gilbert, 2016).

Approaching health risks in terms of probabilities of future harm is aligned with the quantification of modern everyday life (Espeland & Stevens, 2008). It values numbers that turn common domains of life into abstract entities that only experts can formulate, thanks to their training and access to relevant data. Such quantification of possible adverse health outcomes creates a specific way of knowing while assuming a shared cognitive system across all segments of society. However, as stated by Espeland and Stevens (2008), "an ethics of quantification should investigate how the world is made by measures, but should strongly reject any conceit, scientific or otherwise, that measurement provides privileged or exclusive access to the real" (p. 432). Quantification procedures imply by definition a simplification of reality or a decontextualization, with research conducted in laboratories or based on a limited number of factors. These procedures do not account for the complexity of undesirable events as they occur in everyday life. Hence, probabilities constantly clash with real-life experiences. Numbers produced by abstract systems remain opaque to a majority of people (Giddens, 1991), including members of the public but often also experts and professionals, especially when they are outside of their zone of competence.

Efforts to control risks through quantification, often associated with a zero-risk narrative promoted by prevention advocates, are regularly challenged by individual and collective events. First, counterevidence, when a less likely event occurs, contributes to undermining the relevance of formal risk knowledge and indicates that risks provide only partial access to reality. Second, adverse events reveal that beyond the promises of risk management, uncertainty remains omnipresent since an important number of situations are not amenable to calculations, such as in the case of emerging threats (the COVID-19 pandemic or environmental exposures). Third, people are more and more aware that the existence of formal risk knowledge does not systematically equate with risk reduction since conflicting interests might impact its production and circulation, as revealed by controversies, notably those echoed in media channels.

I was particularly interested in how, depending on their position and social circumstances, social actors praise, challenge, complement, or manipulate tools offered by probabilistic thinking. I showed that in real-life circumstances, people, as professionals or citizens, rely on local and embodied knowledge, which helps them relate the abstract idea of risk to their social contexts. Health risks are reinterpreted within these contexts, encompassing elements—for example, senses, past occurrences, and relations—on which individuals have a more concrete hold. When people use their own observations or hints to understand risks, they may complement but also question standardized measures. They reflexively define their own exposure to risk amidst contradictory sources of information (Giddens, 1990). Or, as proposed by the process of individualization

(Beck, 1992) encouraging them to making their own decisions, they act as autonomous citizens weighing conflictual injunctions.

On another note, the coexistence of different ways of knowing about risks reflects the ongoing discussion between research paradigms, which define what counts as knowledge. The dominant position of natural and positivist-oriented science has been challenged over the past decades. Some experts, rather oblivious to the controversies associated with their findings and propositions, remain convinced that this is the best way to prevent future harm. They trust quantitative methodologies controlling for possible factors of 'noise' diverting from the observation of a 'pure' phenomenon, therefore approached outside of real-life circumstances or without paying attention to social factors. This implies for them that a cognitive model of risk, based on probabilities, is preferable to other forms of knowledge and that risk numeracy should be reinforced in society. However, claims that formal risk knowledge is superior to any other form of knowing can better be held when one is distant from concrete decisions and is not personally involved. This distance is seen as a guarantee of objectivity and reason; at the same time, it is often associated with a depreciation of alternative views on risk and uncertainty. It can be considered as a strategy to not question one's self-identity as an expert, who has been 'trained for certainty' according to Atkinson (1984). Besides, this identity has been forged over a long socialization and is often associated with prestige and resources.

However, this position is challenged by alternative models of what counts as knowledge or by the qualitative culture of risk analysis advocated by Jasanoff (1993). The ability to reframe an issue from another person's perspective can indeed lead some to revise their initial judgments. I heard a local pediatrician state that he used to consider parents hesitant toward vaccines 'mentally retarded' (sic). However, he admitted that once he started listening to their concerns, his perception shifted: "After a few years, I became more interested because I realized that these people were much more vigilant when it came to health than the average person" (Deml et al., 2020, p. 112949).

Real-life situations reveal that risk numeracy does not solve the challenges associated with the application of abstract knowledge to concrete individual circumstance, including for medical doctors (Wegwarth &

Gigerenzer, 2018). While formal knowledge is important, it provides only a partial reading of the issues under consideration. This is why empirical findings suggest that in many instances, both professionals and members of the public combine formal and experiential knowledge. Intuition, experiences, and moral convictions are often used by members of the public, professionals, and policy-makers alike when they have to make risk decisions.

In addition to the coexistence of these different forms of knowledge, significant challenges are associated with the processing of large amounts of information available on risks. The assumption that knowing is better than not knowing reflects the high symbolic value of formal knowledge in modern societies (Heimer, 2012). However, as well illustrated by COVID-19 infodemic, the growing amount and rapid circulation of risk knowledge generates important difficulties. Modern media accelerate the diffusion of alternative forms of understanding, including conspiracy theories. Their presence, far from being new since rumors are typical in unsettled times, is reinforced by the viral nature of social media. This massive circulation of knowledge contributes to feed speculations about institutions' potential hidden agendas, but it might also echo instances of previous poor performance or communication of public health agencies. Efforts put into place by officials to counter these alternative narratives—like the material developed by the World Health Organization to respond to the COVID-19 infodemic—suggest enduring power dynamics that aim at maintaining the dominant position of science and expertise.

Conflicts and alliances across multiple forms of knowledge reveal the political processes through which risks are considered acceptable, or not, by individuals in their different social roles (M. Douglas, 1985). Furthermore, the empirical elements I discussed in this chapter contribute to question the opposition between scientific knowledge on the one hand, and uncertainty and ignorance on the other hand. The diffusion of constant doubt and reflexivity as central features of modern societies (Beck, 1992; Giddens, 1990) are indeed aligned with scientific thinking itself. Risk, as a tool for danger management, settled at a time, in the mid-twentieth century, when the authority of science was little challenged. Amid top-down relations, the trust of the public was often taken for granted. However, a few decades later, the challenges and shortcomings of formal risk knowledge currently question the authority of science in these matters.

When people challenge formal risk knowledge promoted by health institutions, they more broadly question their authority. Historically, natural and medical sciences prevailed over social sciences. In the context of health risks, epidemiological and biomedical approaches continue to be dominant, as observed in the management of the COVID-19 pandemic. However, it can be claimed that social sciences have played a major role in the development of reflexivity across society over the past decades by revealing the limits of science in its production and circulation. They analyze the shortcomings of expertise by paying attention to concerns ignored by dominant institutions, but central to some people's experiences.

These shortcomings call for the integration of additional elements in the thinking developed around risks. In that respect, the social science contribution is progressively better acknowledged. In addition, the promotion of participatory formats in medical and public health decision bodies, more often including patients and citizens, reflects a redistribution of power, progressively unsettling the authority of positivist science through the inclusion of other forms of knowledge. Efforts dedicated to the anticipation of harm contribute to these new dynamics.

References

Akinbi, A., Forshaw, M., & Blinkhorn, V. (2021). Contact tracing apps for the COVID-19 pandemic: A systematic literature review of challenges and future directions for neo-liberal societies. *Health Information Science and Systems, 9*(1), 18. https://doi.org/10.1007/s13755-021-00147-7

Akrich, M. (2010). From communities of practice to epistemic communities: Health mobilizations on the internet. *Sociological Research Online, 15*(2), 17.

Armstrong, D. (1995). The rise of surveillance medicine. *Sociology of Health & Illness, 17*(3), 393–404.

Armstrong, D. (2014). Actors, patients and agency: A recent history. *Sociology of Health & Illness, 36*(2), 163–174. https://doi.org/10.1111/1467-9566.12100

Armstrong, N. (2019). Navigating the uncertainties of screening: The contribution of social theory. *Social Theory & Health, 17*(2), 158–171. https://doi.org/10.1057/s41285-018-0067-4

Armstrong, N., & Eborall, H. (2012). *The sociology of medical screening. Critical perspectives, new directions*. Wiley-Blackwell.

Atkinson, P. (1984). Training for certainty. *Social Science and Medicine, 19*(9), 949–956.

Attwell, K., Hannah, A., & Leask, J. (2022). COVID-19: Talk of 'vaccine hesitancy' lets governments off the hook. *Nature, 602*(7898), 574–577. https://doi.org/10.1038/d41586-022-00495-8

Aven, T., & Bouder, F. (2020). The COVID-19 pandemic: How can risk science help? *Journal of Risk Research, 23*, 1–6. https://doi.org/10.1080/13669877.2020.1756383

Aven, T., & Renn, O. (2009). On risk defined as an event where the outcome is uncertain. *Journal of Risk Research, 12*(1), 1–11.

Beck, U. (1992). *Risk society. Towards a new modernity*. Sage. [1986: first edition in German *Risikogesellschaft*].

Beck, U. (1999). *World risk society*. Polity Press.

Berger, P., & Luckmann, T. (1991 [1966]). *The social construction of reality. A treatise in the sociology of knowledge*. Penguin Books.

Bernstein, P. L. (1996). *Against the gods. The remarkable story of risk*. John Wiley & Sons.

Bickerstaff, K. (2004). Risk perception research: Socio-cultural perspectives on the public experience of air pollution. *Environment International, 30*(6), 827–840. https://doi.org/10.1016/j.envint.2003.12.001

Bogner, A. (2015). Decision-making under the condition of uncertainty and non-knowledge: The deliberative turn in genetic counselling. In M. Gross & L. McGoey (Eds.), *Routledge international handbook of ignorance studies* (pp. 199–205). Routledge, Taylor & Francis Group.

Bourdelais, P. (2003). *Les épidémies terrassées*. Editions de la Martinière.

Bourrier, M., Brender, N., Burton-Jeangros, C., & (Éds.). (2019). *Managing the global health response to epidemics: Social science perspectives*. Routledge.

Bourrier, M., & Burton-Jeangros, C. (2014). Ni malades, ni en bonne santé. *Socio-anthropologie, 29*, 7–12.

Brown, P. (1987). Popular epidemiology: Community response to toxic waste-induced disease in Woburn, Massachusetts. *Science, Technology, & Human Values, 12*(3/4), 78–85.

Brown, P. (1992). Popular epidemiology and toxic waste contamination: Lay and professional ways of knowing. *Journal of Health and Social Behaviour, 33*, 267–281.

Brown, P. (2021). *On vulnerability: A critical introduction* (1st ed.). Routeldge.

Browner, C. H., & Press, N. (1996). The production of authoritative knolwedge in American prenatal care. *Medical Anthropology Quarterly, 10*(2), 141–156.

Burton-Jeangros, C. (2004). *Cultures familiales du risque*. Economica.

Burton-Jeangros, C. (2011). Surveillance of risks in everyday life: The agency of pregnant women and its limitations. *Social Theory & Health, 9*(4), 419–436. https://doi.org/10.1057/sth.2011.15

Burton-Jeangros, C. (2019). Epidemics and risk communication why are lessons not learned? In M. Bourrier, N. Brender, & C. Burton-Jeangros (Eds.), *Managing the global health response to epidemics: Social science perspectives*. Routledge.

Burton-Jeangros, C., Aceti, M., Chappuis, P., Tsantoulis, P., & Hurst, S. (submitted). Bénéfices et limites de l'évaluation des risques de cancer par l'oncogénétique prédictive Une étude par forums citoyens. *Santé Publique*.

Burton-Jeangros, C., Cavalli, S., Gouilhers, S., & Hammer, R. (2013). Between tolerable uncertainty and unacceptable risks: How health professionals and pregnant women think about the probabilities generated by prenatal screening. *Health, Risk & Society, 15*(2), 144–161. https://doi.org/10.1080/13698575.2013.771737

Bury, M. (1997). *Health and illness in a changing society*. Routledge.

Caiata-Zufferey, M., Pagani, O., Cina, V., Membrez, V., Taborelli, M., Unger, S., Murphy, A., Monnerat, C., & Chappuis, P. O. (2014). Challenges in managing genetic cancer risk: A long-term qualitative study of unaffected women carrying BRCA1/BRCA2 mutations. *Genetics in Medicine*. https://doi.org/10.1038/gim.2014.183

Callon, M., Lascoumes, P., & Barthe, Y. (2001). *Agir dans un monde incertain. Essai sur la démocratie technique*. Seuil.

Caron-Flinterman, J. F., Broerse, J. E. W., & Bunders, J. F. G. (2005). The experiential knowledge of patients: A new resource for biomedical research? *Social Science & Medicine, 60*(11), 2575–2584.

Castel, R. (1983). De la dangerosité au risque. *Actes de la recherche en sciences sociales, 47–48*, 119–127.

Chiolero, A., Paccaud, F., Aujesky, D., Santschi, V., & Rodondi, N. (2015). How to prevent overdiagnosis. *Swiss Medical Weekly*. https://doi.org/10.4414/smw.2015.14060

Clarke, A. E., Mamo, L., Fishman, J. R., Shim, J. K., & Fosket, J. R. (2003). Biomedicalization: Technoscientific transformations of health, illness and US biomedicine. *American Sociological Review, 68*(2), 161–194.

Conrad, P., Bandini, J., & Vasquez, A. (2016). Illness and the Internet: From private to public experience. *Health: An Interdisciplinary Journal for the Social Study of Health, Illness and Medicine, 20*(1), 22–32. https://doi.org/10.1177/1363459315611941

Crawford, R. (1980). Healthism and the medicalization of everdyday life. *International Journal of Health Services, 10*(3), 365–388.

Debergh, M. (2022). *La santé sexuelle à l'épreuve du local. Une ethnographie féministe en Suisse romande*. PhD in sociology, University of Geneva.

Dedieu, F., & Jouzel, J.-N. (2015). Comment ignorer ce que l'on sait? La domestication des savoirs inconfortables sur les intoxications des agriculteurs par les pesticides. *Revue française de sociologie, 56*(1), 105–133. https://doi.org/10.3917/rfs.561.0105

Deml, M. J., Buhl, A., Notter, J., Kliem, P., Huber, B. M., Pfeiffer, C., Burton-Jeangros, C., & Tarr, P. E. (2020). 'Problem patients and physicians' failures': What it means for doctors to counsel vaccine hesitant patients in Switzerland. *Social Science & Medicine, 255*, 112946. https://doi.org/10.1016/j.socscimed.2020.112946

Doron, J.-P. (2016). The experience of risk. In A. Burgess, A. Alemanno, & J. Zinn (Eds.), *Routledge handbook of risk studies*. Routledge, Taylor & Francis Group.

Douglas, K. M., Uscinski, J. E., Sutton, R. M., Cichocka, A., Nefes, T., Ang, C. S., & Deravi, F. (2019). Understanding conspiracy theories. *Political Psychology, 40*(S1), 3–35. https://doi.org/10.1111/pops.12568

Douglas, M. (1985). *Risk acceptability according to the social sciences*. Routledge & Kegan Paul.

Douglas, M. (1990). Risk as a forensic resource. *Daedalus, 119*(4), 1–16.

Earnshaw, V. A., Eaton, L. A., Kalichman, S. C., Brousseau, N. M., Hill, E. C., & Fox, A. B. (2020). COVID-19 conspiracy beliefs, health behaviors, and policy support. *Translational Behavioral Medicine, 10*(4), 850–856. https://doi.org/10.1093/tbm/ibaa090

Epstein, S. (1998). *Impure science: AIDS, activism, and the politics of knowledge* (Reprint). University of California Press.

Erikson, K. (1990). Toxic reckoning: Business faces and a new kind of fear. *Harvard Business Review, 90*(1), 118–126.

Espeland, W. N., & Stevens, M. L. (2008). A sociology of quantification. *European Journal of Sociology, 49*(3), 401–436. https://doi.org/10.1017/S0003975609000150

Ewald, F. (1986). *L'Etat providence*. Bernard Grasset.

Eysenbach, G. (2009). Infodemiology and infoveillance: Framework for an emerging set of public health informatics methods to analyze search, communication and publication behavior on the Internet. *Journal of Medical Internet Research, 11*(1), e11. https://doi.org/10.2196/jmir.1157

Fernandez Pinto, M. (2017). To know or better not to. Agnotology and the social construction of ignorance in commercially driven research. *Science & Technology Studies, 30*, 53. https://doi.org/10.23987/sts.61030

Foucault, M. (1989 [1966]). *Les mots et les choses: Une archéologie des sciences humaines*. Gallimard.

Foucault, M. (2004 [1978]). *Sécurité, territoire, population*. Gallimard [u.a.].

Franks, B., Bangerter, A., Bauer, M. W., Hall, M., & Noort, M. C. (2017). Beyond "monologicality"? Exploring conspiracist worldviews. *Frontiers in Psychology, 8*, 861. https://doi.org/10.3389/fpsyg.2017.00861

French, M., & Mykhalovskiy, E. (2013). Public health intelligence and the detection of potential pandemics: Public health intelligence and the detection of potential pandemics. *Sociology of Health & Illness, 35*(2), 174–187. https://doi.org/10.1111/j.1467-9566.2012.01536.x

Frickel, S., & Vincent, M. B. (2007). Hurricane Katrina, contamination, and the unintended organization of ignorance. *Perspectives on Hurricane Katrina, 29*(2), 181–188. https://doi.org/10.1016/j.techsoc.2007.01.007

Fujimura, J. H., & Holmes, C. J. (2019). Staying the course: On the value of social studies of science in resistance to the "post-truth" movement. *Sociological Forum, 34*, 1251–1263. https://doi.org/10.1111/socf.12545

Furedi, F. (2009). Precautionary culture and the rise of possibilistic risk assessment. *Erasmus Law Review, 2*(2), 197–220.

Giddens, A. (1990). *The consequences of modernity*. Polity Press.

Giddens, A. (1991). *Modernity and self-identity in the late modern age*. Polity Press.

Gigerenzer, G. (2008). *Gut feelings: The intelligence of the unconscious*. Penguin Books.

Gilbert, C. (2016). Revisiter les risques à l'aune de la sécurité ordinaire—Postface. In S. Becerra, M. Lalanne, & J. Weisbein (Eds.), *Faire face aux risques dans les sociétés contemporaines* (pp. 267–274). Octarès éditions.

Gillespie, C. (2015). The risk experience: The social effects of health screening and the emergence of a proto-illness. *Sociology of Health & Illness, 37*(7), 973–987. https://doi.org/10.1111/1467-9566.12257

Glik, D. C. (2007). Risk communication for public health emergencies. *Annual Review of Public Health, 28*(1), 33–54. https://doi.org/10.1146/annurev.publhealth.28.021406.144123

Green, J., Draper, A., & Dowler, E. A. (2003). Short cuts to safety: Risk and « rules pf thumb » in accounts of food choice. *Health, Risk & Society, 5*(1), 33–52.

Gross, M., & McGoey, L. (2015). *Routledge international handbook of ignorance studies*. Routledge, Taylor & Francis Group.

Halloy, A., Simon, E., & Hejoaka, F. (2022). Defining patient's experiential knowledge: Who, what and how patients know. A narrative critical review. *Sociology of Health & Illness, 45*, 405–422. https://doi.org/10.1111/1467-9566.13588

Hammer, R. P., & Burton-Jeangros, C. (2013). Tensions around risks in pregnancy: A typology of women's experiences of surveillance medicine. *Social Science & Medicine, 93*, 55–63. https://doi.org/10.1016/j.socscimed.2013.05.033

Heimer, C. A. (2012). Inert facts and the illusion of knowledge: Stategic uses of ignorance in HIV clinics. *Economy and Society, 41*(1), 17–41.

Henderson, L., & Hilton, S. (2018). The media and public health: Where next for critical analysis? *Critical Public Health, 28*(4), 373–376. https://doi.org/10.1080/09581596.2018.1482663

Heyman, B., Henrisken, M., & Maughan, K. (1998). Probabilities and health risks: A qualitative approach. *Social Science & Medicine, 47*(9), 1295–1306.

Heymann, D. (2006). SARS and emerging infectious diseases: A challenge to place global solidarity above national sovereignty. *Annals of the Academy of Medicine, Singapore, 35*(5), 350–353.

Hofmann, B. (2016). Disease, illness, and sickness. In *The Routledge companion to philosophy of medicine*. Routledge. https://doi.org/10.4324/9781315720739.ch2

Höppner, C., Whittle, R., Bründl, M., & Buchecker, M. (2012). Linking social capacities and risk communication in Europe: A gap between theory and practice? *Natural Hazards, 64*(2), 1753–1778. https://doi.org/10.1007/s11069-012-0356-5

Jasanoff, S. (1993). Bridging the two cultures of risk analysis. *Risk Analysis, 13*(2), 123–129. https://doi.org/10.1111/j.1539-6924.1993.tb01057.x

Jonas, H. (1990). *Le principe de responsabilité: Une éthique pour la civilisation technologique*. Les Editions du Cerf.

Jurich, E. K. (2021). 'Do you think this is normal?': Risk, temporality, and the management of children's food allergies through online support groups. *Health, Risk & Society, 23*(3–4), 128–142. https://doi.org/10.1080/13698575.2021.1914824

Kenen, R. (1996). The at-risk health status and technology: A diagnostic invitation and the « gift » of knowing. *Social Science & Medicine, 42*(11), 1545–1553.

Klepac, P., Kucharski, A. J., Conlan, A. J., Kissler, S., Tang, M., Fry, H., & Gog, J. R. (2020). Contacts in context: Large-scale setting-specific social mixing matrices from the BBC Pandemic project [Preprint]. *Epidemiology*. https://doi.org/10.1101/2020.02.16.20023754

Krause, N. M., Freiling, I., Beets, B., & Brossard, D. (2020). Fact-checking as risk communication: The multi-layered risk of misinformation in times of COVID-19. *Journal of Risk Research, 23*(7–8), 1052–1059. https://doi.org/10.1080/13669877.2020.1756385

Lakoff, A. (2017). *Unprepared: Global health in a time of emergency*. University of California Press.

Lakoff, A. (2022). Preparedness indicators: Measuring the condition of global health security. *Sociologica, 21*, 25–43. https://doi.org/10.6092/ISSN.1971-8853/13604

Leiss, W. (1996). Three phases in the evolution of risk communication practice. *The Annals of the American Academy of Political and Social Science, 545*, 85–94.

Lupton, D. (2016). *The quantified self: A sociology of sel-tracking*. Polity.

Markens, S., Browner, C. H., & Preloran, H. M. (2010). Interrogating the dynamics between power, knowldege and pregnant bodies in amniocentesis decision making. *Sociology of Health and Illness, 32*(1), 37–56.

Moodie, R., Stuckler, D., Monteiro, C., Sheron, N., Neal, B., Thamarangsi, T., Lincoln, P., & Casswell, S. (2013). Profits and pandemics: Prevention of harmful effects of tobacco, alcohol, and ultra-processed food and drink industries. *The Lancet, 381*(9867), 670–679. https://doi.org/10.1016/S0140-6736(12)62089-3

Mooney, S. J., & Pejaver, V. (2018). Big data in public health: Terminology, machine learning, and privacy. *Annual Review of Public Health, 39*(1), 95–112. https://doi.org/10.1146/annurev-publhealth-040617-014208

Moore, W. E., & Tumin, M. M. (1949). Some social functions of ignorance. *American Sociological Review, XIV*, 787–795.

Nathanson, C. A. (1996). Disease prevention as social change: Toward a theory of public health. *Population and Development Review, 22*(4), 609–637.

Nerlich, B., & Koteyko, N. (2012). Crying wolf? Biosecurity and metacommuncation in the context of the 2009 swine flu pandemic. *Health and Place, 18*, 710–717.

Nicholls, S. G. (2013). Standards and classification: A perspective on the 'obesity epidemic'. *Social Science & Medicine, 87*, 9–15. https://doi.org/10.1016/j.socscimed.2013.03.009

Norddal, G. A., Wifstad, Å., & Lian, O. S. (2022). 'It's like getting your car checked': The social construction of diabetes risk among participants in a population study. *Health, Risk & Society, 24*(3–4), 93–108. https://doi.org/10.1080/13698575.2022.2028742

O'Donnell, S. (2015). Changing social and scientific discourses on type 2 diabetes between 1800 and 1950: A socio-historical analysis. *Sociology of Health & Illness, 37*(7), 1102–1121. https://doi.org/10.1111/1467-9566.12292

O'Malley, P. (2016). Governmentality and the analysis of risk. In A. Burgess, A. Alemanno, & J. Zinn (Eds.), *Routledge handbook of risk studies*. Routledge, Taylor & Francis Group.

OECD. (2003). *Emerging risks in the 21st century. An agenda for action*. OECD.

Ogden, J. (1995). Psychosocial theory and the creation of the risky self. *Social Science and Medicine, 40*, 409–415.

Owens, K. (2022). The passivists: Managing risk through institutionalized ignorance in genomic medicine. *Social Science & Medicine, 294*, 114715. https://doi.org/10.1016/j.socscimed.2022.114715

Peretti-Watel, P., & Moatti, J.-P. (2010). Renoncer à l'homo medicus pour mieux comprendre les conduites à risque. *Contacts santé, 23*, 52–53.

Pinto, M. F. (2015). Tensions in agnotology: Normativity in the studies of commercially driven ignorance. *Social Studies of Science, 45*(2), 294–315. https://doi.org/10.1177/0306312714565491

Popay, J., & Williams, G. (1996). Public health research and lay knowledge. *Social Science & Medicine, 42*(5), 759–768. https://doi.org/10.1016/0277-9536(95)00341-X

Prior, L. (2003). Belief, knowledge and expertise: The emergence of the lay expert in medical sociology. *Sociology of Health and Illness, 25*(3), 41–57.

Proctor, R., & Schiebinger, L. L. (Eds.). (2008). *Agnotology: The making and unmaking of ignorance*. Stanford University Press.

Pulido, C. M., Villarejo-Carballido, B., Redondo-Sama, G., & Gómez, A. (2020). COVID-19 infodemic: More retweets for science-based information on coronavirus than for false information. *International Sociology, 35*(4), 377–392. https://doi.org/10.1177/0268580920914755

Rabeharisoa, V., Moreira, T., & Akrich, M. (2014). Evidence-based activism: Patients', users' and activists' groups in knowledge society. *BioSocieties, 9*(2), 111–128. https://doi.org/10.1057/biosoc.2014.2

Rayner, S. (2012). Uncomfortable knowledge: The social construction of ignorance in science and environmental policy discourses. *Economy and Society, 41*(1), 107–125. https://doi.org/10.1080/03085147.2011.637335

Renn, O. (2008). *Risk governance: Coping with uncertainty in a complex world.* Earthscan.

Rhodes, T., & Lancaster, K. (2021). Excitable models: Projections, targets, and the making of futures without disease. *Sociology of Health & Illness, 43*(4), 859–880. https://doi.org/10.1111/1467-9566.13263

Rhodes, T., & Lancaster, K. (2022). Making pandemics big: On the situational performance of Covid-19 mathematical models. *Social Science & Medicine, 301*, 114907. https://doi.org/10.1016/j.socscimed.2022.114907

Rhodes, T., Lancaster, K., Lees, S., & Parker, M. (2020). Modelling the pandemic: Attuning models to their contexts. *BMJ Global Health, 5*(6), e002914. https://doi.org/10.1136/bmjgh-2020-002914

Rose, N. (2013). Personalized medicine: Promises, problems and perils of a new paradigm for healthcare. *Procedia - Social and Behavioral Sciences, 77*, 341–352. https://doi.org/10.1016/j.sbspro.2013.03.092

Roslyng, M. M., & Eskjær, M. F. (2017). Mediatised risk culture: News coverage of risk technologies. *Health, Risk & Society, 19*(3–4), 112–129. https://doi.org/10.1080/13698575.2017.1286298

Sacks, G., Swinburn, B. A., Cameron, A. J., & Ruskin, G. (2018). How food companies influence evidence and opinion – straight from the horse's mouth. *Critical Public Health, 28*(2), 253–256. https://doi.org/10.1080/09581596.2017.1371844

Saukko, P. (2018). Digital health - a new medical cosmology? The case of 23andMe online genetic testing platform. *Sociology of Health & Illness, 40*(8), 1312–1326. https://doi.org/10.1111/1467-9566.12774

Scammell, M. K., Senier, L., Darrah-Okike, J., Brown, P., & Santos, S. (2010). Tangible evidence, trust and power: Public perceptions of community environmental health studies. *Social Science and Medicine, 68*, 143–153.

Schuetz, A. (1953). Common-sense and scientific interpretation of human action. *Philosophy and Phenomenological Research, 14*(1), 1–38. https://doi.org/10.2307/2104013

Short, J. F. (1984). The social fabric at risk: Toward the social transformation of risk analysis. *American Sociological Review, 49*(December), 711–725.

Skolbekken, J.-A. (2008). Unlimited medicalization? Risk and the pathologization of normality. In A. Petersen & I. Wilkinson (Eds.), *Risk, health and vulnerability* (pp. 16–29). Routledge.

Slovic, P. (1992). Perceptions of risk: Reflections on the psychometric paradigm. In S. Krimsky & D. Golding (Eds.), *Social theories of risk* (pp. 117–152). Praeger.

Slovic, P. (2000). *The perception of risk*. Earthscan.

Stern, A. M., & Markel, H. (2004). International efforts to control infectious diseases, 1851 to the present. *JAMA, 22*(29), 1474–1479.

Swidler, A., & Arditi, J. (1994). The new sociology of knowledge. *Annual Review of Sociology, 20*, 305–329.

Timmermans, S., & Buchbinder, M. (2010). Patients-in-waiting: Living between sickness and health in the genomics era. *Journal of Health and Social Behavior, 51*(4), 408–423. https://doi.org/10.2307/20798303

Tversky, A., & Kahneman, D. (1974). Judgment under uncertainty: Heuristics and biases. *Science, 185*, 1124–1131.

Vargas, N., Mora, G. C., & Gleeson, S. (2023). Race and Ideology in a pandemic: White privilege and patterns of risk perception during COVID-19. *Social Problems, 70*(1), 219–237. https://doi.org/10.1093/socpro/spab037

Vassy, C., Dingwall, R., & Murcott, A. (2007). Comment analyser l'absence d'anticipation des risques? Le cas de la canicule de 2003 en France. *Sociologie et sociétés, 39*(1), 161–179.

Vernazza, P., & Bernard, E. (2016). HIV is not transmitted under fully suppressive therapy: The Swiss Statement – eight years later. *Swiss Medical Weekly, 146*, w14246. https://doi.org/10.4414/smw.2016.14246

Wang, Y., McKee, M., Torbica, A., & Stuckler, D. (2019). Systematic literature review on the spread of health-related misinformation on social media. *Social Science & Medicine, 240*, 112552. https://doi.org/10.1016/j.socscimed.2019.112552

Washer, P. (2010). *Emerging infectious diseases and society*. Palgrave Macmillan.

Weber, M. (1963 [1919]). *Le savant et le politique* (10–18 ed.). Union Générale d'Éditions [1917 original version in German *Wissenschaft als Beruf* und 1919 *Politik als Beruf*].

Weber, M. (1964 [1904]). *L'éthique protestante et l'esprit du capitalisme: Suivi d'autres essais*. Plon. [1905 original version in German *Die protestantische Ethik und der Geist des Kapitalismus*].

Wegwarth, O., & Gigerenzer, G. (2018). The barrier to informed choice in cancer screening: Statistical illiteracy in physicians and patients. In U. Goreling & A. Mehnert (Eds.), *Psycho-oncology*. Springer.

Weir, L., & Mykhalovskiy, E. (2007). The geopolitics of global public health surveillance in the twenty-first century. In A. Bashford (Ed.), *Medicine at the border: Disease, globalization and security, 1850 to the present* (pp. 240–263). Palgrave Macmillan UK. https://doi.org/10.1057/9780230288904_13
Welch, G. (2011). *Overdiagnosed. Making people sick in the pursuit of health.* Beacon Press.
Wigginton, B., & Lafrance, M. N. (2014). 'I think he is immune to all the smoke I gave him': How women account for the harm of smoking during pregnancy. *Health, Risk & Society, 16*(6), 530–546. https://doi.org/10.1080/13698575.2014.951317
World Economic Forum. (2023). *The Global Risks Report 2023* (18th ed.). WEF.
Wynne, B. (1996). May the sheep safely graze? A reflexive view of the expert-lay knowledge divide. In S. Lash, B. Wynne, & B. Szerszynski (Eds.), *Risk, environment and modernity: Towards a new ecology* (pp. 44–83). Sage.
Zinn, J. O., & Schulz, M. (2024). Rationalization, enchantment, and subjectivation – lessons for risk communication from a new phenomenology of everyday reasoning. *Journal of Risk Research, 27*(2), 295–312. https://doi.org/10.1080/13669877.2024.2328195

3

Anxiety, Fear, and Panic: The Role of Emotions in Prevention

Introduction

The idea of risk emphasizes control over adverse situations and is expected to eliminate fear in human activities. As a consequence, from the perspective of formal risk management, emotions such as anxiety, fear, and panic are associated with disorder and considered to bias decisions. In risk communication, messages typically struggle with the balance to find between avoiding to induce fear and eliciting confidence. However, emotions are inevitable in contemporary environments focused on risk reduction since they reflect people's engagement with their own life and with others. This was formulated in an early social science definition of risk: "A hazard, in our parlance, is a threat to people and to what they value (property, environment, future generations) and risk is a measure of hazard" (Kates & Kasperson, 1983, p. 7029). For social scientists, the expression of emotions is framed by the sociocultural environment, which defines what people should be afraid of and which fears are legitimate. Within the prevailing cultural background of pessimism and anxiety, I claim that a number of negative emotions profoundly shape social interactions and views on what ought to be done to avert danger across society.

C. Burton-Jeangros, *Experiences of Health Risks*, Critical Studies in Risk and Uncertainty, https://doi.org/10.1007/978-3-031-65377-3_3

I examine here the multiple, often ambivalent, roles that emotions play in the anticipation of the future. In contrast to the formal risk management, which approaches them as a source of bias against rational action, I suggest that anxiety, fear, and panic significantly shape the experiences and strategies developed around risk. They are important in the elaboration of meanings, and I discuss how they guide actions related to the mitigation of harm in society in both official and lay responses. Indeed, emotions seem to contribute to tackling intangible situations of risk and uncertainty, as these regularly escape the control promised by responses solely based on reason or cost–benefit trade-offs.

This chapter then discusses the role of emotions in health risk prevention, as they are raised by screening and surveillance measures, encouraging constant monitoring to initiate early action. At the same time, across a number of health domains, emotions are often amplified by professionals and policy-makers when they strive to engage the public in preventive actions. Hence, while risk management aims at removing fear, I show that dealing with risk often involves emotional components, which can contribute to unsettle experiences of health.

After describing how emotions are approached through a sociological lens, I discuss how fear is addressed in social theories dedicated to risks, from risk perception research to the description of the modern culture of fear. Before turning to empirical illustrations, I also introduce a few elements related to emotions in sociology of health. The second part of the chapter presents the contrasting ways in which emotions associated with risks—ranging between anxiety and panic—have been addressed in research focused on health risks.

Social Sciences Approach to Emotions and Risks

Sociology of Emotions

Early sociologists analyzed the process of modernization with a focus on the growing importance of secular rationality (Shilling, 2002), which attributed a marginal role to emotions in society. More serious attention has been given to emotions only since the 1980s, as indicated by reviews on the anthropology of emotions (Lutz & White, 1986) and sociology of emotions (Thoits, 1989). Next to interpretative approaches to social reality, scholars have introduced emotion in the analysis of human experience to move beyond the dominant focus on cognitive and rational-economic motivations for action (Lutz & White, 1986). Considering that affective components are inherent to human action, they foster a sociological analysis of emotions, since according to Barbalet (2002), "no action can occur in a society without emotional involvement" (p. 2). Emotions contribute to creating bonds between individuals and their context, as well as connections among individuals. Hochschild's concept of emotion work proposes that the expression of emotions is context dependent: "we assess the 'appropriateness' of a feeling by making a comparison between feeling and situation, not by examining the feeling in abstract" (1979, p. 560). Therefore, beyond being physiological responses, emotions are socially elaborated.

Among the vast range of emotions that can be observed, some are considered to play a more crucial role in the organization of society. Fear, which is closely related to the anticipation of danger, is one of them. According to Bericat (2016), people express fear when they think that their interests are threatened. He considers that fear embraces a range of more or less intense feelings between worry, anxiety, and panic or even horror. Others make a distinction between fear and anxiety, suggesting that fear is directed toward a definite object, while anxiety is more diffuse and not specifically attached to any specific situation (Starkstein, 2018).

At the macro level, societies differ in their definitions of appropriate emotional climates. Variations in fears across time and culture described by anthropological and historical research (Bourke, 2006) confirm that "emotional beliefs are both socially acquired and socially structured" (Thoits, 1989, p. 319). Indeed, social contexts define appropriate emotional responses to specific situations; within a range of relevant responses, feeling rules shape what one should and should not feel or express (Hochschild, 1979; Thoits, 1989). Such culturally appropriate emotional climates and reactions are acquired via socialization and reproduced through interactions (Bericat, 2016), including display rules, defining expectations toward others.

At the micro level, individuals react to the circumstances they encounter in prevailing emotional climates while taking into account their own resources and relationships (Bericat, 2016). When facing danger, resources are indeed important. Confidence toward the future is frequent among those who have power and material resources (Francis, 2007; Turner & Stets, 2006), while fear and anxiety are more prevalent among those who feel powerless (Kemper, 1991). In addition, emotions are regulated by social interactions: "Fear often emerges in social contexts, not as a mere individual reaction to a threat, but as the result of an intersubjective experience" (Bericat, 2016, p. 504). Relations can thus either reinforce or value some emotional responses while attenuating or rejecting others. As a consequence, individuals engage in emotion work when they try "to change in degree or quality an emotion or feeling" (Hochschild, 1979, p. 559), making their reactions adequate in their specific context.

Taking emotions seriously implies to reject the assumption that fact-based rationality is the unique yardstick to be used for action and that emotions introduce biases in decisions (Bandes, 2008). Rather, following Nussbaum (2001) suggesting that emotions reveal judgments about what matters for individuals, they should be considered useful. First they help to sort out massive amounts of information circulating about a specific issue: "they help us to interpret, organize and prioritize the information that bombard us" (Bandes, 2008, p. 422). Second the emphasis on 'judgements of value' adds that emotions reveal the social meanings attached to specific situations (Kahan, 2008). Hence "fear is the appropriate and accurate judgment for someone who values her or another's well-being in the face of an impending threat to it" (Kahan, 2008, p. 109).

I thus want to stress here that, from a sociological perspective, emotions are inherent to social action, reflect normative expectations, and facilitate social interactions. Their appreciations in the social theories of risk are introduced next.

Social Theories of Risk and Emotions

With his early statistical work on mortality records in England in the seventeenth century, Graunt explicitly stated that scientific knowledge could eliminate fear of disease and death (Doron, 2009). Indeed, formal risk management defines fear and panic in negative terms as irrational and emotional reactions are devalued compared to actions aligned with scientific knowledge and analytical reasoning. Early on, formal risk knowledge strived to alleviate fear by framing possible futures and guiding action according to cost–benefit analyses. Expressions of anxiety, fear, and panic are therefore considered sources of disorder due to emotional biases introduced in decisions. The very success of the notion of risk explains this strong discrediting of fear; indeed, the antinomy between knowledge and fear is central in modern culture: "rationality and emotion are mainly understood as a duality of two factors which exclude themselves mutually" (Zinn, 2006, p. 2). Approached as physiological responses, emotions were also long associated with nature and passivity, thus opposed to the active stance of action based on reason and science.

However, from its very beginning, risk perception research has provided insights into the importance of anxiety and fear in people's reactions to danger. The first empirical findings in the 1970s emphasized two main dimensions of risk perceptions, namely, emotion and cognition (Slovic, 2000). The first dimension, named 'dread', is explicitly related to emotions with risks characterized by being uncontrollable, potentially catastrophic, dangerous to future generations, and involuntary. It contrasted with the second dimension, named 'unknown risk', bringing together cognitive features encompassing risks that are chronic, unknown to those exposed, delayed, and new. While initially discarded, the positive role of emotions in decisions, through the provision of hints in complex and uncertain situations, has been later acknowledged in that research tradition (Slovic et al., 2004).

According to social theorists of risk, against the assumptions of risk management, anxiety, fear, and panic have not been alleviated in the risk society but rather to the contrary (Lupton, 2013b). Indeed, Beck (1992) emphasized the association between an increasing awareness of risk and the exacerbation of anxiety. The diminishing trust in institutions' capacity to protect individuals from risks induced by the very development of modern society reinforces such an emotional climate. Furthermore, globalization accompanied by a growing awareness of systemic and uncertain threats (Giddens, 1990) has been adding to a general sense of vulnerability. Wilkinson (2001) emphasized that the diffusion of anxiety did not target specific events, rather it was reinforced by overall feelings of uncertainty about the future. Preferring the concept of fear, Furedi (1998), in the '*Culture of Fear*', and Bauman (2006), in '*Liquid Fear*', described the main features of what they considered to be a new cultural context. It is important to stress that these notions emerged at a time when vulnerability was increasingly emphasized in relation to growing social inequalities at the turn of the twenty-first century, with welfare systems failing to protect individuals against new social risks (Castel, 2003). Together, these changes led to a shift from the overall optimism of the post-1945 decades to a currently dominant pessimistic approach to the future at both the individual and collective levels.

This negative stance has been reinforced by the proliferation of expert statements warning against potential danger, the constant expansion of insurance schemes to anticipate adverse outcomes, and the permanent focus of the media on danger. Together, they challenge people's confidence in the regular course of their life. Indeed, they are regularly reminded by institutions and the media that they might be exposed to adversity and should thus consider themselves vulnerable (Bauman, 2006). Dominant safety preoccupations have transformed many activities—previously considered banal and unexceptional—into potential risks. In the words of Bauman (2006), efforts to manage risks paradoxically fuel the gap between actual dangers, many of which are framed and mitigated in modern societies, and fears expressed among the population. In other words, there can never be enough safety since preoccupations with risks continue to emphasize the marginal danger left unattended. In his description of worst-case thinking, Clarke (2006) suggested that "what really makes something worst is not the event itself but what people *think about* the event" (p. 16, author's emphasis). The idea of risk is exactly about this: it frames a specific way to think about a potential situation. Constant anticipation of what could happen has been triggered by formal risk management, expecting individuals in their different positions—as professionals or as citizens—to be attentive to their action of today at the light of what could happen later.

At the same time, unexpected circumstances, in which the course of things did not follow expert scenarios, keep questioning the capacity to control the future promised by risk calculations. The shortcomings of science supported the development of alternative approaches such as the precautionary principle, which is more popular in Europe and calls for anticipation in the absence of knowledge to prevent the unexpected (Ewald, 1996). At approximately the same time, in the United States, possibilistic thinking gained in popularity in some organizational settings or individual decisions, leading to anticipating the worst case characterized by the absence of control (Clarke, 2006). These approaches, which depart from formal risk management, are likely to fuel emotional responses. Indeed, members of the public experience a widespread "sentiment of being *susceptible* to danger, a feeling of insecurity and vulnerability" (Bauman, 2006, p. 3). The anticipation of risk, leading to the formulation of different scenarios, encourages individuals to make decisions while anticipating the consequences of their decisions. This contributes to feed emotional responses since "the possibility of choosing creates anxiety, given that the outcomes of choices are often unknown" (Starkstein, 2018, pp. 273–274). Overall, the prevailing values of autonomy and individual freedom are likely to exacerbate anxiety feelings in society (Rebughini, 2021). However, these general statements need to be nuanced since, as discussed in Chap. 6, anxiety and feelings of vulnerability are not homogenous across social categories (Finucane et al., 2000).

In addition to declining trust in experts and institutions, individual anxiety might further be fed by the awareness of "human company as a source of existential insecurity" (Bauman, 2006, p. 132). For example, in the context of the COVID-19 pandemic or environmental change, risks induced through the actions of others were emphasized. Suspicion toward others is amplified when individuals are asked to contribute to the prevention of danger by signaling potentially dangerous individuals or behaviors, as in the case of warnings in public transport. These schemes not only reinforce the idea that danger is everywhere but also imply that others should be systematically distrusted (as further explored in Chap. 5).

In social theories of risk, the role of emotions has thus been progressively integrated (see also Lupton, 2013b; Zinn, 2006, 2016). Furthermore, other theoretical frameworks addressing the gap between emotional reactions and actual danger should be mentioned here, including the literature on fear of crime and moral panic. Both are interested in the mismatch observed between the statistical framing of an issue and different groups' interpretations. Fear of crime relates to the gap between statistical measures of crime risks and fears expressed in the population, that is, evaluations of potential victimization (Warr, 2000). It is observed that nondominant groups—for example, elderly people and women—express more fear of crime. The distinction made between fear for self and fear for others (adults for their children and for their elderly parents) also situates such feelings of vulnerability within networks of relations (Kimber et al., 2018). Some groups regularly report elevated feelings of vulnerability or are constructed by others as vulnerable and in need of protection, next to appraisals encompassing emotional dimensions beyond actual danger.

The moral panic literature refers to the, often short-lived, discrepancy between an actual danger and sudden social attention tending to exaggerate its extent: "At times, substantial numbers of the members of societies are subject to intense feelings of concern about a given threat which a sober assessment of the evidence suggests is either nonexistent or considerably less than would be expected from the concrete harm posed by the threat" (Goode & Ben-Yehuda, 1994, p. 149). It has been considered that mass media play a particularly significant role in these mechanisms as they contribute to generating indignation (Walsh, 2020). These processes are nowadays exacerbated by social media through the viral diffusion of concerns: "By inflating the visibility of inflammatory content, social media mobilize animosity toward common enemies and transform uneasy concern into full-blown panic" (p. 845). Developed outside the social theories of risk, both of these perspectives suggest that interpretations of danger that do not align with statistical measures are colored by emotions, as indicated by the terms "fear" of crime and moral "panic". They have in common an emphasis on the framing of an issue by groups of actors, as a social process leading to interpretations of risks amplifying danger beyond probabilities.

Emotions and risks thus appear as close companions across these various theoretical contributions. The former seem to be an inevitable component of risk, as they play an important role in society and in social interactions. I also consider important to emphasize the currently high prevalence of negative emotions, over positive ones, a process fed by successive global crises of different nature.

Emotions in Sociology of Health

Emotions have been little integrated into sociology of health and illness and then mostly approached through the lens of stress and mental health (Francis, 2007). Their neglect reflects here again the uneasiness toward domains outside a reason-based approach. Such a narrow focus contributes to restrict attention given to interactions that exist between individuals, in their embodiment, and their social contexts. Nevertheless, two aspects are worth considering here. First, some authors suggest that emotions might represent the missing link between the biological and social dimensions of health, second the absence of emotions in scholarship is interpreted as a sign of the strength of medical preferences for organic explanations and technical solutions.

As regard the first aspect, several authors see emotions as a possible connector between the biological or organic and the social realities. Francis (2007) emphasized this connection by stating that: "emotion is the touchstone for overcoming the rationalist dualism of Western thought, in which self and society are viewed as irreductibly separate and biology is unconnected to social structure" (p. 591). Emotions are expressed through bodily reactions that relate individuals to their immediate environment and to others (Powell & Gilbert, 2008). Hence, emotional reactions feed intersubjectivity through expressions of the body displayed according to socially shared rules (Francis, 2007). Such an understanding encourages us to take emotions seriously.

Turning to the second aspect, debates about the origins of stress and anxiety, as mental health issues, persist among scholars of different disciplines. While the medical approach is focused on their biological roots, sociologists proposed that they are the result "of a generalized experience of powerlessness in the face of adverse existential conditions" (Freund, 1990, p. 463), since status insecurity generates existential anxiety. People occupying less valued positions in social hierarchies, based on their social class, gender, age, or race, would feel powerless and thus experience negative emotional states. By contrast, those occupying valued positions in society tend to deny such experiences of powerlessness and their associated emotional reactions. They thus reproduce social hierarchies by imposing a form of social control through the definition of proper reactions toward adversity. The recurrent downplaying of 'emotions' in the public by some risk experts and medical practitioners reflects such power relationships: "Having one's feelings ignored or termed as irrational is the analogue of having one's perceptions invalidated (Hochschild 1983:173)" (in Freund, 1990, p. 466).

Not considering the social circumstances underlying emotional expressions reflects medicine's tendency to neglect the role of factors situated outside of the organic body. Following the development of psychoanalysis at the beginning of the twentieth century, psychiatry has endorsed chemical solutions, including an expanding use of anxiolytics over the twentieth century (Starkstein, 2018). "Overmedicalization is a logical extension of the rationalization of Western thought, in which the individual self is seen as prior to and separate from society. As such, causes of emotional distress are seen as located in the biology of the individual, in, for example, the levels of the neurotransmitter serotonin" (Francis, 2007, p. 594). This individualized and biological approach makes it impossible to consider the expression of emotions within social environments.

These elements confirm the poor consideration of emotions, reduced to their physiological expression, by a number of disciplines. It results from the overwhelming role attributed to reason and cognition and is associated with limited attention given to bodies and emotions. A social science perspective offers, however, valuable insights about the expressions of fear, anxiety, and stress which encourage to situate emotions within people's social circumstances. As I show in the second part of the chapter, emotions are omnipresent around risk prevention interventions; it is thus important to examine their ambivalent roles.

Anxiety, Fear, Panic, and Health Risks

Against this background showing that emotions are progressively being integrated into the theorization of risks and health, I now turn to how fear in its various forms has been approached across a number of health risks. The multifaceted presence of fear across different prevention domains reveals the ambivalence induced by emotions. First, I discuss how the failing body, as emphasized by secondary prevention aimed at detecting early signs of disease, is a source of anxiety and creates demands for reassurance from the public. Second, I review how some primary prevention campaigns deliberately summon emotions to induce behavioral change by eliciting fear. Third, turning to the concept of panic, I address how emerging or expanding risks, when perceived as out of control by experts, generate official overreactions or moral panics aimed at overcoming the assumed passivity of the public. Finally, the debated role of the media in inducing panic, notably around infectious diseases, is addressed. This diversity of aspects already indicates the omnipresence of emotions in a field that tends to avoid them.

The Failing Body: Anxiety as a Consequence of Routine Preventive Measures

The articulation of risk and anxiety around health issues was emphasized early on, for example, by Rose et al. (2008 [1992]), who acknowledged that prevention can produce anxiety. Social science research conducted around the development of routine preventive measures reveals recurrent tensions between the anticipation of risks, anxiety, and a need for reassurance.

Currently, a number of screening procedures, such as cervical cancer, breast cancer, prenatal testing, hypertension, for example, are routinely performed on healthy individuals to determine their likelihood of developing a disease. Screening is valued in society as a means to anticipate disease and is promoted by expert guidelines (Armstrong & Eborall, 2012). People usually undergo these procedures upon the invitation of professionals or at their own initiative in the case of opportunistic screening programs. In all cases, screening produces new personal knowledge: individual results are assessed against average values, which are used to establish the division between normal and pathological results.

Nevertheless, regardless of the results, the process of screening inevitably makes people aware of potential risks related to their health condition. This has been emphasized in the very common measurement of child development according to a standardized growth chart: this routine procedure keeps drawing mothers' attention to potential deviations, which are then labeled abnormalities (Olin Lauritzen & Sachs, 2001). Prenatal screening, including regular tests over the pregnancy course, also questions pregnant women's confidence by constantly exposing them to further results that might show flaws in themselves or their child to be (Thomas et al., 2017). A gynecologist-obstetrician interviewed in Switzerland observed that the provision of information on risk is 'double-edged' (Burton-Jeangros et al., 2013, p. 7): while it confirms the proper course of a pregnancy, it induces expectations for risk control and certainty that are in reality difficult to reach. In this study, we indeed identified a category of women whose experience of pregnancy was characterized by constant worry: they tended to expect something bad to happen, talking about the viability of their fetus, the risks of miscarriage, fetal anomalies, or premature delivery even though none of the tests they had performed could substantiate their anxiety (Hammer & Burton-Jeangros, 2013).

The medical surveillance of risks encourages mothers to assess the risks associated with their daily routines, and some expressed anxiety about being personally responsible to avoid harm. A mother reported to me that to mitigate the risk of mad cow disease in the late 1990s, she was using agar–agar as a replacement for gelatin, but without being sure that this strategy would protect her family (Burton-Jeangros, 2004). Discovering the impossibility of finding definite answers to potential adverse consequences of mundane actions while pregnant also produces discomfort. The uncertainty regarding the potential harm of cosmetic use or some specific foods makes pregnant women the sole arbitrator of their decisions. Their constant attention to averting risks—promoted by routine pregnancy medical surveillance—turned for some into a never-ending quest for safety that proves unreachable (Burton-Jeangros, 2011).

Their preoccupation is aligned with the precautionary principle, suggesting that the absence of evidence is not proof of the absence of danger.

The potential harms of expanding genetic testing are being discussed (Sturdy, 2022). While knowing about actionable risks can support preventive measures, some of the observed genetic variations are not related to any possible preventive measures, such as being at increased risk for Alzheimer's disease. In addition, even when measures can be taken, just knowing about one's own increased risk is a source of concern. The people we convened in forums to discuss developments in oncogenetics frequently raised concerns about the emotional cost of this knowledge. Knowing one to be at risk was considered a source of stress, and several participants suggested that it could in itself reduce their quality of life (Burton-Jeangros et al., submitted). This was also observed in the context of a mass screening program on abdominal aortic aneurysm in Sweden, with members of the targeted population of men aged over 65 reporting ambivalent feelings toward knowing more about their personal risk (Hansson et al., 2012). These statements suggest that more knowledge can therefore prove counterproductive.

In contrast, screening results of individuals situated in the 'normal' group—that is, below the threshold defining a pathological value—represent the optimal scenario for both professionals and people under surveillance. In a study on screening for prediabetic status, when no risk was identified, "participating in a screening induced positive emotions of relief and reassurance" (Norddal et al., 2022, p. 12). Some participants valued the knowledge they had gained, feeling empowered by their 'body audit', comparing it to 'getting your car checked'. Reassurance was defined as having gained more years of good health and as having a favorable impact on quality of life.

Overall, anxiety generated by screening procedures modifies the relationships between screened individuals and professionals. Indeed, when confronted with uncertainty, both doctors and patients are inclined to ask for more tests, with the hope of gaining more knowledge and hence reducing anxiety. This came up in studies on cervical cancer screening (Burton-Jeangros et al., 2015), pregnancy surveillance (Hammer & Burton-Jeangros, 2013), and prediabetic screening (Norddal et al., 2022). In ethnographic observations of sexual health consultations, professionals agreed to perform an HIV test, even when unwarranted, merely to reassure a client (Debergh, 2022). Gynecologists-obstetricians have also been shown to use more technical procedures—such as an additional morphologic ultrasound—to better evaluate Down syndrome risks when the initial statistical values were borderline. Nevertheless, additional information still did not provide certainty about the absence of chromosomal anomalies (Cavalli, 2014a). These illustrations reveal the new dynamics induced by efforts to identify risks: they create demands for reassurance since expectations for certainty induced among the public by risk thinking contribute to anxiety.

Indeed, techniques and instruments used to measure risks, as intangible elements beyond individuals' actual perceptions, feed the increasing gap between people's conditions and their appreciation of them. As a result, preventive procedures have been associated with the emergence of the "worried well", referring to individuals a priori in good health but who do not feel confident in their own perceptions or in the absence of any symptom. Following Bauman (2006), the idea of being susceptible to risk could thus be sufficient to generate a sense of vulnerability. General practitioners interviewed in the early 1990s already reported on this category of "worried well" who end up overusing preventive services (Williams & Calnan, 1994). Such anxiety inflation among some patients, who are more often situated in privileged social positions, has gained traction, and the term is now being used by clinicians and in United Kingdom health policy-making (Gray et al., 2020). Criticizing the inadequate use of the term and its judgmental connotations, this article published in the *British Journal of General Practice* emphasizes the central role that general practitioners can play in providing reassurance. At the same time, their capacity to provide such reassurance is continuously jeopardized by risk thinking, which exposes professionals to litigation in cases of improper anticipation (Manaï et al., 2010). In other words, health anxiety supports public demands for additional medical procedures and testing; in parallel the logic of risk with its expectations of control makes it difficult for professionals to dismiss these demands.

In summary, the implementation of biomedical risk management involves eliciting emotions in the context of routine screening for the early detection of disease or malformation. In policy debates and media reports, these are typically depicted as a problem since such expressions of anxiety run against 'feeling rules' promoted by risk management, which foremost see emotions as a source of bias. However, I claim that the accumulation of risk knowledge is profoundly ambivalent: while providing a rational means to gain control and thus discard fears, it simultaneously generates negative feelings by continuously eliciting multiple scenarios for the future without providing certainty and confidence. This might contribute to explain why, despite improving health levels in the United States, measures of well-being declined in the general population (Schnittker, 2009). I consider that constantly monitoring individual risks through routine screening not only impacts sociocultural expectations of health, but more largely promotes a sense of inherent vulnerability.

Governing Through Fear

In addition to these 'unexpected' emotions resulting from the very attempt to control risks, they are in some cases used as a resource by health promoters. Scholars, notably ethicists and social scientists, continue to debate the pros and cons of using fear to encourage people to change their behaviors across prevention campaigns dedicated to smoking, obesity, cancer, road accidents, HIV/AIDS, or COVID-19 (Fairchild et al., 2015, 2018; Guttman & Lev, 2021).

In a context saturated with information and diversifying communication channels, health education campaigns starting in the last decades of the twentieth century explicitly turned to marketing strategies to gain public attention (Bunton et al., 1995). The use of threatening public information has been particularly popular in Anglo-Saxon countries since the early twentieth century in the United States to promote hygiene, vaccination, and the prevention of sexually transmitted diseases (Fairchild et al., 2018). More recently, it has been especially prominent in smoking prevention, at the international level with the massive adoption of scary images on cigarette packages since the 2000s, supported by the European Office of the World Health Organization. However, in the context of the HIV/AIDS epidemic, the use of fear has been debated since the early 1980s, and a rather consensual position prevailed about avoiding messages inducing fear with the explicit intention to limit stigmatization (Fairchild et al., 2018). Nevertheless, in the context of the COVID-19 pandemic, a number of reports have again indicated the use of fear in different contexts to support the public's adherence to official recommendations. These included images of mass burials, COVID-19 patients suffering in an overloaded hospital, sounds from a popular horror movie in relation to a local curfew, or people acting as ghosts to pass on messages (Guttman & Lev, 2021). This recurrence of fear-arousal messages confirms the intuitive attractiveness of scare tactics among some prevention experts (Fairchild et al., 2015; Kok et al., 2018; Peters et al., 2013).

Appeals to fear reveal their conviction that emotions are appropriate for modifying behaviors among passive and apathetic people (Lupton, 2013b): "These discourses suggest that such individuals should be frightened, anxious, disgusted or ashamed, for it is these emotions that will impel them into rational action: that is, taking steps to avoid contracting illness or disease" (p. 644). Indeed, across a number of campaigns, some specialists believe that scare tactics are justified for generating emotional reactions. This was, for example, the case for smoking prevention in Australia, with public health professionals prone to recommending fear tactics (David Hill et al., 1998, p. 7). Confirming the importance of emotions in decision-making, Chapman and Coups (2006) concurred that "emotions are more immediate precursors of decision than are calculations of the risk probabilities and severity" (p. 88) and suggested that interventions appealing to emotions are more likely to influence behaviors than those based on statistical measures of risk.

Even though it has been debated since the 1950s (Janis & Feschbach, 1953), scare tactics in public health continue to be both used and challenged. Some suggest that fear and worry are a proper avenue for health education (Hammond et al., 2004; Lemal & Van den Bulck, 2010; Witte & Allen, 2000). Others claim that it does not impact practices in the expected manner (Earl & Albarracín, 2007; Peters et al., 2013). The controversy is illustrated by the accumulation of reviews and meta-analyses, as well as debates among researchers through comments on each other's conclusions in scientific journals. The debate concerns the size of the impact and the different factors implicated in behavioral change. Critics claim that the effects are limited and that the evidence is biased by publication politics which prioritize research showing effects over studies producing null findings (Kok et al., 2018). Those who question this strategy also emphasize that appeals to fear among individuals who have a low sense of self-efficacy, hence those who do not believe they can actually change their behavior, might backfire. Indeed, these people are likely to discard the message and could even be reinforced in their practices: "warning labels on packs of cigarettes seem ill-advised. They may in fact increase smoking among smokers who derive self-esteem from their identity as a smoker" (Peters et al., 2013, p. S27). In that case, prevention would be counterproductive, with consequences standing in contradiction with its goals.

The controversy is further fueled by a number of methodological concerns, notably as regards measurement of change in behaviors. First, the impact is usually assessed as an intention to change rather than actual change. Second, the effects of scary messages over time are not followed-up and these could be short term and lead to denial or annoyance later (Guttman & Lev, 2021; Hastings & Stead, 2004). In other words, some scholars believe that the complex relationship between perception and behavior is not sufficiently addressed in these strategies. In addition, randomized controlled trials, the gold standard format for such research, are difficult to implement to assess messages that are already largely disseminated in society (Kok et al., 2018), or when conducted in experimental settings, they are not paying attention to people's actual circumstances in daily life (Hastings & Stead, 2004). In other words, these strategies are not sufficiently attentive to real-life conditions of behavioral change.

Some scholars have also raised a number of ethical concerns in this context (Guttman & Salmon, 2004; Guttman & Lev, 2021; Brookes & Harvey, 2015; Oxman et al., 2022). First, deliberately raising anxiety and worry in the public is deemed ethically problematic since it infringes on individual autonomy. At the same time, individual freedom must be compounded by the risks that people can impose on others with their decisions, such as through smoking or avoiding vaccination (Oxman et al., 2022). In the context of the COVID-19 facemask measures, these authors discussed how messages can be situated on a continuum from information to coercion, with intermediate stages of recommendation, persuasion, and manipulation. The emphasis on using evidence to formulate messages was particularly weak in the early stage of the COVID-19 pandemic and the associated infodemic (Stolow et al., 2020). Second, the impact of scare tactics is not uniform across the population. Considering the importance of self-efficacy in behavioral change, scare tactics are more likely to benefit more privileged people while inducing denial and/or distress among those in less favorable social positions (Hastings & Stead, 2004). Thus, scare tactics might contribute to increasing health inequalities across social groups (see Chap. 6). Third, campaigns using emotions impact relations across social groups. Appeals to emotion navigate between fear and disgust toward those who do not endorse healthy lifestyles recommendations (Fairchild et al., 2015; Lupton, 2013b). By generating such emotions, campaigns establish divisions between people and reinforce the stigmatization of those who do not comply with recommendations (Thompson et al., 2009) (see Chap. 5).

Fourth, fear appeals should also question the agenda of policy-makers encouraging such tactics. In the context of preventing sexually transmitted infections in young adults in the United Kingdom, Gagnon stated that "fear is inherently political since it is deployed by the state with the clear objective of penetrating the collective and personal domains to manage/govern the population and their sexual behaviors" (2010, p. 249). This suggests that manipulation might be considered justified in some circumstances to support some policy goals. However, campaigns exaggerating risks to induce behavioral change do not match people's experiences. Thus, official agencies can be perceived as dishonest and hypocritical in their selection of some risks, in some population groups, while leaving aside other forms of danger (Hastings & Stead, 2004). Ultimately, scare tactics might contribute to undermining the trust in authorities criticized for using manipulative strategies. Such diminished trust in institutions might have broader political consequences.

This ongoing controversy about the explicit use of fear tactics reveals the ambivalence generated by emotions in public health spheres. Fear tactics, as top-down approaches using psychological models to alter risk behaviors, are considered legitimate by some to reach health promotion goals. However, in addition to having undue consequences that run against prevention, they can contribute to making policy-makers appear deceitful and patronizing (Deml et al., 2019; Wynia, 2006).

Panic in Public Health

The social amplification of risk theory aims at addressing the gap between technical risk assessments and social reactions to these evaluations (Kasperson et al., 1988). It pays attention to the circulation of information about risks in society, and its potential distortion, in which emotions might play a role. In this section, I first discuss how experts mobilize emotions in their own appreciation of health threats and in their anticipation of general public reactions. Then, I raise instances of risk attenuation by professionals, when danger is minimized to avoid emotional responses in the public, and risk amplification, when danger is exaggerated behind the statistical measures to capture public attention. The section thus shows how professional communication navigates between contradictory intentions, on the one hand, the attention given to protecting the public from undue anxiety and, on the other hand, the desire to activate social reactions when danger is considered high.

Enduring Bias Toward Public Panic

Beyond the explicit use of fear discussed above, social science research has addressed the role of emotions in expert judgments with the idea of panic. According to Fairchild and Merritt Johns (2015), there is an enduring conviction among policy-makers in the United States that the public is prone to panic. They explain this as a legacy of LeBon contagion theory, suggesting that emotion in times of crisis is rapidly circulating from person to person and leading to social chaos due to irrational and selfish behaviors. This belief in the likelihood of the public to panic has been shown to be common among social science scholars, officials, and leaders, as well as in the media and fiction (Clarke, 2002; Quarantelli, 2001; Sheppard et al., 2006). Hence, panic reactions in front of danger seem intuitively appealing to many people.

At the individual level, panic refers to episodes of acute anxiety, labeled 'panic attack' or 'panic disorder' (Sheppard et al., 2006). In the context of crises or emerging risks, it is usually approached at the collective level with assumptions about how people are likely to behave under such circumstances. Clarke (2002) mentions the Oxford English Dictionary definition of panic as an "excessive feeling of alarm or fear… leading to extravagant injudicious efforts to secure safety" (p. 21). Next to the widespread devaluation of emotions discussed above, panic is typically associated with negative characteristics such as being irrational, antisocial, impulsive, nonfunctional, maladaptive, and inappropriate (Quarantelli, 1954). Attributes of reckless action and selfishness are common (Clarke, 2002). Panic is thus related to social disorder associated with a breakdown of social relations, possibly generating further danger (Clarke & Chess, 2008).

Scholars describe officials' enduring belief in panic, as apparent in policy-making around infectious diseases and bioterrorism. Preparedness, scenarios, and large-scale exercises entail measures to anticipate panic and to control psychological reactions. This focus of experts on panic is, however, criticized: "planners and policymakers sometimes act as if the human response to threatening conditions is more dangerous than the threatening conditions themselves" (Clarke & Chess, 2008, p. 994). This was indeed the case with the World Health Organization efforts to counter the adverse effects of the infodemic generated by the COVID-19 pandemic.

Against these pervasive assumptions, empirical evidence shows that panic is rare. It was not observed in situations as diverse as the sarin attacks in the Tokyo metro in 1995, the 9/11 World trade center evacuation, the anthrax attacks in September 2001, the subway bombing in London in 2005 (Sheppard et al., 2006), and Three-mile island accident in 1979 (Glass & Schoch-Spana, 2002). Research on reactions to fire over more than 100 years has reached similar conclusions (Johnson, 1987). In all these situations, contrary to expectations, disorder or chaos was absent, while cohesion and cooperation prevailed among those affected (Clarke, 2002; Quarantelli, 2001). Such statements do not imply that fear was absent: "while strong emotions were experienced, these did not lead to maladaptative behavior" (Quarantelli, 2001, p. 8). Scholars conclude that rather than generating reckless and individualistic responses, disasters reinforce the social fabric: "people are naturally social, and calamities often strengthen social bonds" (Clarke, 2002, p. 25). These findings suggest that, in crises and disruptive events, socialization and moral obligations might predominate over selfish considerations or chaos (Clarke & Chess, 2008). Instead, they emphasize the profound influence of social order on individuals (Sheppard et al., 2006).

One is then left to wonder why is public panic so often expected? This could reflect the strength of the economic model of human behavior, suggesting that individuals are rational and selfish (Frey et al., 2010). This model, focused on individual behaviors, leads to the assumption that crisis situations should generate selfish responses from people focused on protecting their own interest. From another perspective, Clarke (2002) considers that the 'myth of panic' might serve institutional interests since it provides an official justification to retain some information on the presumption that this information might have detrimental consequences. By maintaining the idea of a gap between rational experts and disproportionately emotional reactions among the public, these authors suggest that panic can be considered "an approach that advances the power of those at the top of organizations" (Clarke & Chess, 2008, p. 944).

The elements I discussed in this section imply that it is important to question official assumptions regarding the propensity of the public to panic. Their recurrence might reflect the extent of anxiety among professionals having to manage crises rather than a largely observed social phenomenon.

Avoiding Public Overreactions

Case studies describe how, in some circumstances, officials deliberately do not share some information to not create overreactions in the public. In a French study on the late acknowledgment of the adverse consequences of diethylstilbestrol (DES) on reproductive capacity, doctors justified the absence of communication to potentially concerned women by their wish to avoid overreactions (Fillion & Torny, 2016). They assumed that concerned patients had to be protected, anticipating their negative emotional reactions. Another instance of professional emotional work is offered in the work of Cavalli (2014b) on the management of information by gynecologists-obstetricians when discussing low probability risks related to prenatal screening. In the past, doctors collected and interpreted screening data without necessarily sharing their aims and results with their patients. However, current bioethical standards require health professionals to inform their patients about the procedures they undertake. They are aware that the provision of information about potential risks can generate anxiety, while it is frequently undue when test results show that an individual's values do not show a personal elevated risk. Therefore, some doctors acknowledged that they preferred to limit the amount of information before performing screening, hoping that the results would show that the pregnant woman was not at risk and thus avoided inducing anxiety. In those cases, silence was deemed acceptable against the expected negative emotional impact of the information if it was delivered.

In the context of re-emerging infectious diseases, the gap between experts and the public regarding emotional reactions was also discussed. An analysis of H1N1 governmental material in Australia suggests that official documents reflect how public health policy is navigating between generating compliance with official measures while not creating overreactions. For officials, pandemic control would be "a remarkably delicate art of styling communication to promote compliance but without producing either complacency or panic" (Davis et al., 2011, p. 915). It appears that on many occasions, experts do not trust people, often evoking their emotional responses. This might contribute to explaining the lack of engagement with local populations in the resolution of crises. This was observed in the context of Ebola management when teams deployed from international agencies often did not engage with local populations (Bourrier, 2019). In the United States, Lakoff (2017) emphasized the absence of the public in national preparedness exercises. In Switzerland, the work performed by the Swiss National COVID-19 Scientific Task Force—in which I participated—has also long remained confined to experts with limited participation from civil society representatives.

The repetition of this divide keeps suggesting that the public should not be trusted under conditions of danger and stress, while professionals would present appropriate reactions. Nevertheless, I consider that the bad press of emotions in risk management might backfire at the end of the day in their relationships with the public. Indeed, when officials keep relevant information from people, to protect these against their own emotions, they stand in contradiction with the ethical principles of autonomy and transparency in modern democracies. Common assumptions about the public as passive, "only capable of under- or over-reacting" (Davis et al., 2011, p. 917), should be challenged. They also stand in contradiction with participatory procedures that should be valued when dealing with emerging threats.

Risk Amplification or Public Health Moral Panics

In other public health domains, official reactions have been analyzed as being biased by experts' fears toward specific issues: "Panic is an attribution that is almost exclusively applied when looking down at people who do not occupy positions of power or authority. However, panic can also be seen by looking up, although it is rare that anyone does so" (Clarke & Chess, 2008, p. 1006). Such panic from experts would be more likely in times of intense scrutiny from the media on official responses. This was, for example, observed in the aftermath of the Katrina hurricane in New Orleans, when officials disseminated misrepresentations of the local populations accusing lower class residents of looting instead of paying attention to the impact of the catastrophe on the more deprived groups of the population. In this section, I discuss instances of risk amplification suggesting that moral panics might indeed result from overreactions among experts, often reinforced by the media. They concern situations considered preoccupying, often referred to as an epidemic curve of increasing cases and/or reflecting out-of-control issues; they include notably obesity, tobacco, re-emerging infectious diseases, and bioterrorism.

In the context of re-emerging infectious diseases, it has been suggested that official overreactions were observed in a number of crises, from the swine flu controversy of the late 1960s to decisions to vaccinate millions of people against smallpox after the 2001 anthrax episode (Fairchild & Merritt Johns, 2015). In the management of A(H1N1), Margaret Chan WHO's director-general initially decided against declaring a pandemic in May 2009 "because the very term 'pandemic' was feared to trigger global panic" (Gilman, 2010); however, she still declared it a pandemic a few weeks later. Bonneux and Van Damme (2011) suggested that the WHO response at that time was prompted by the general culture of fear and worst-case thinking, aligned with the importance of a preemptive strike: "The pandemic policy was never informed by evidence, but by fear of worst-case scenarios" (p. 539). The alarmism of the World Health Organization in 2009 was criticized once the virus turned out to have limited consequences (Bourrier et al., 2019). According to Gilman (2010), the WHO reaction was stirred by the anticipation of an upcoming major epidemic with the associated expertise: "Such a situation stirs many qualities and emotions to create an illness, not in the sense of inventing it, but in the sense of shaping our experience of it. The 2009 H1N1 influenza turned out not to be the equivalent to 1918. Yet the power of the threat and the attendant panic was [sic] real" (p. 1867). I personally witnessed the importance of emotions while attending virtual meetings of the Swiss National Science COVID-19 Task Force in Spring 2020 when epidemiological evidence was interpreted in completely contrasting ways by different members of the group, some calling for a total long-term lockdown while others were being much more lenient. In all these cases, the preparedness and training of experts did not eliminate the role of emotions in decisions related to unprecedented and little documented events.

Over the past two decades, a number of social scientists have discussed how emotions pervade obesity prevention as a major public health concern. A body of literature discusses the gap between scientific evidence and official positions on obesity, tainted by emotions, and the role of the media in this amplification of obesity risks. In the context of noncommunicable diseases, obesity has become a major target for public health, initially in Anglo-Saxon countries but more recently turning into a major global health concern due to its international expansion. Epidemiological data showing the increase in obesity rates in affluent countries over the past decades have led some specialists to formulate alarmist predictions using a vivid vocabulary depicting the "epidemic" of obesity and comparing its impact on society to the threat of terrorism. For example, a leading official in the United States (formerly Attorney General Richard Carmona) referred to the obesity epidemic as "a 'terror within' and predicted that it would 'dwarf 9/11' in terms of human suffering" (Patterson & Johnston, 2012, p. 273). Major public health agencies such as the

Centers for Disease Control and Prevention in the United States and the World Health Organization contributed to this framing with documents that "frequently sensationalize obesity as a disease to be feared, and a contagion to avoid" (p. 282). These positions are not aligned with scientific evidence, since findings now suggest that obesity rates might be stabilizing or even declining in Western countries (Bombak, 2014). However, it has been observed that some specialists dismiss or challenge the facts that counter their own position on the obesity issue and new results are "met with surprise, doubt, and resistance" (Bombak, 2014, p. 516). By adhering to a model emphasizing individual responsibility, they also dismiss alternative environmental explanations and social determinants of health. These reactions have been attributed to the 'fat phobia' of some experts.

Such framing by scientists was extended by the media, whose attention to obesity increased in parallel to the developments of research in that domain (Saguy & Riley, 2005). Empirical analyses suggest that obesity risks are dramatized and sensationalized in mass media coverage (Monaghan et al., 2019; Patterson & Johnston, 2012), associated with a moral panic dynamic or even a fat panic. Terms connotated with fear and anxiety are typically used, including "epidemic", "war", or "time bomb". As an illustration, the Daily Mail in 2015, a popular UK tabloid, reported as a headline the words of the Chief Medical Officer who declared that women's obesity was "as dangerous as terror threat" (Monaghan et al., 2019, p. 4). Like scientists, media outlets have shown limited endorsement of newer epidemiological findings. Media were considered so biased that specialists published a piece in the Lancet, a leading medical journal, asking the media to tone down their reporting (Flint et al., 2018).

It is considered that overreactions toward obesity have been supported by a range of "obesity epidemic entrepreneurs", including scientists, officials, and the media, whose intention was clearly to capture society's attention about this new risk. In addition to fear, other emotions, such as shame and disgust, have also been commonly convened (Lupton, 2013a), which further color reactions toward obese people. These elements reflect an elite-engineered moral panic around obesity, which is considered by some to be out-of-control and inducing social disorder that needs to be averted. In this case, moral judgments and fear have contributed to shaping interpretations of epidemiological evidence (Bombak, 2014).

With these examples, I wanted to illustrate the extent of alarmist reactions by public health officials across different domains. These reactions confirm that anxiety, fear, and panic are also omnipresent in expert risk thinking. They often remain implicit or invisible since they are considered not legitimate. At the same time, some note that panic can serve the interest of experts: "invoking panic is an extremely effective means of riveting public attention at a moment of risk and uncertainty, securing resources, and establishing or challenging policies aimed at either control or amelioration of the disease or other threats we associate with social disorder" (Fairchild & Merritt Johns, 2015, p. 178). These considerations further confirm the important role of emotions in the regulation of risk in society.

Media Studies on Fear and Panic Related to Health Crises

It has long been considered that traditional media coverage of health risks does not align with their statistical distribution. For the media, crises, risks, uncertainties, and emotions are good ingredients for capturing public attention. Indeed, as I show in this section, their reporting has been considered a key element in moral panics (Ingraham & Reeves, 2016).

At the beginning of the twenty-first century, scholars started to discuss the ambivalent role of the media in outbreaks of infectious diseases. Indeed, the acceleration of public health crises has mirrored the radical expansion of mass media since the 1980s (Washer, 2010). Infectious disease outbreaks seem particularly prone to media amplification, as recently observed in the context of the COVID-19 pandemic. Such amplification is, however, rather recent. In the early phases of the HIV/AIDS epidemic, the long-term silence of the mass media was emphasized (Herzlich & Pierret, 1989; Ungar, 1998). Media interest in infectious diseases started in the mid-1990s with the reinforcement of re-emerging infectious disease expertise and the dissemination of dramatic scenarios in popular culture through film and fiction writing (Ungar, 1998). While the media remained fairly silent over the first decade of the HIV epidemic, scientists later blamed them for generating undue fear and panic among the population through the reporting of "inaccurate, sensationalized, or misleading stories [...] that are not necessarily the most scientifically significant" (Glik, 2007, p. 42).

As mentioned in Chap. 2, relationships between public health specialists and the media are charged with contrasted agendas and roles. Considered an indispensable partner of official risk communication efforts (Burton-Jeangros, 2019), the media still claim their autonomy. On the one hand, they have a duty to monitor the performance of the government and institutions (Hughes et al., 2006) and thus report on controversies. On the other hand, they do more than reproduce official sources of information since they produce narratives of risk, integrating facts into normative and social contexts (Mairal, 2011). From the perspective of the social amplification of risks, the extent of the dramatization performed by the media continues to be debated (Rossmann et al., 2018).

Efforts have been made to empirically measure media amplification. Media studies typically assess the volume and content of media reports on epidemics. Findings obtained in the pre-COVID-19 period suggest that if the volume of media content generated by infectious diseases is often high, it is usually rather short-lived. Importantly it has been observed that media coverage does not systematically overlap with the number of cases (Brodie et al., 1998; Hilton & Hunt, 2010), that is, media reporting does not simply mirror the increase and subsequent decrease in the number of epidemiological cases. However, a number of media content analyses concluded that their reporting remains factual and neutral (Hilton & Hunt, 2010; Kilgo et al., 2018; Klemm et al., 2016; Vasterman & Ruigrok, 2013). In regard to H1N1, differences were noted between "quality" and "tabloid" papers, with a stronger emphasis on drama and emotions in the latter than in the former (Rossmann et al., 2018). Overall, empirical evidence thus does not support the claims that the media are misrepresenting outbreaks as disproportionately dangerous. Some scholars have concluded that negative emotions related to outbreaks, in the case of H5N1 (Nerlich & Halliday, 2007) or H1N1 outbreaks (Vasterman & Ruigrok, 2013), result from the combined reactions of experts, officials, and journalists, more than from media overreactions in themselves.

However, the role of social media has been appraised differently. A number of authors suggest that they exacerbate collective alarm (Walsh, 2020). Indeed, they contribute to the amount of information shared, and they accelerate the pace of diffusion, while their content remains unfiltered. These supports are not only used by officials and lay individuals but also harnessed by nonhuman sources, with bots generating automated content (Keith Conti et al., 2020). On the one hand, social media channels offer opportunities for those who feel that they lack the means to share their views, particularly to express dissenting positions, and hence are usually loaded with emotions. On the other hand, an analysis of the Centres for Disease Control Facebook page related to the Zika epidemic showed that members of the public blamed the agency for having exaggerated the extent of this epidemic through the media, using a narrative of fear. Some people questioned the collusion between the U.S. Centers for Disease Control and Prevention and Big Pharma, suspecting biases in scientific evidence as a result of economic incentives that together encouraged the purchase of unnecessary vaccines (Laurent-Simpson & Lo, 2019). Such suspicion had been present earlier in the H1N1 pandemic and later in the COVID-19 context, supported by the massive economic benefits of the pharmaceutical industry.

In other words, the media are clearly part of the prevalence of negative emotions related to health risks. However, I showed that they are not solely responsible for generating anxiety and fear since emerging or developing health threats are good candidates for moral panics. A number of moral entrepreneurs converge in producing emotionally and morally laden views, which in turn shape public reactions.

Conclusion

This chapter showed that emotions related to health issues are very present in contemporary contexts as a result of the pervasiveness of risk thinking. Probabilities and epidemiological modeling create possible—more or less likely—futures, most often foreseen on their dark side in terms of upcoming catastrophes, pandemics, accidents, or diseases. The constant projection toward the future brought about by risk thinking expands the sense of personal and collective vulnerability. Acute concerns regarding individual and collective health, as a fundamental condition of social order and functioning, are likely to fuel stress and anxiety. Indeed, I suggest that such fear is exacerbated by the eagerness to gain control over future situations, as promoted by formal risk management. What is new is not the extent of anxiety, since it has been omnipresent in past societies (Giddens, 1991), but rather the fact that it tends to be considered inappropriate.

Nevertheless, against the dominant narrative of control, people remain aware of their still limited capacity to mitigate upcoming danger. Depending on their resources, they are likely to feel more or less vulnerable but also more or less able to respond to the different dangers to which they are exposed (see Chap. 6). These features support the expression of negative emotions, especially since people are frequently reminded of the accumulation of global threats and their individual vulnerability, which unsettle their confidence in the future.

Risks continue to question routines and taken-for-granted reality by forecasting disruption, and they rarely leave people indifferent. Hence, emotions attached to experiences of risk reveal people's commitments to their social world, with others who matter to them and, more broadly, with what they value, as proposed by Kates and Kasperson (1983). Therefore, I claim that people actually engage with risks through emotions associated with embodied experiences: fear and anxiety, but also intuition, pleasure, guilt, and shame—additional emotions addressed in further chapters—which are inevitable components of this engagement. For instance, screening tests are more than information on a physiological parameter; they depict a more or less likely and desirable future. Interpretations of how this imagined future might impact one's social roles and engagements toward others convene emotions beyond cognitive elements. Emotions are particularly important to consider in the interactions occurring between physical and mental health, since they provide a link between feelings of personal vulnerability in health and recurrent references to collective challenges in controlling risks.

Considering the shortcomings of a rational approach to health risks, emotions can thus help people select among massive and contradictory information (Bandes, 2008). Such selection usually serves to confirm their identity through attachment to their loved ones and to social groups who share their interpretations of danger and validate their reactions. At the same time, emotional reactions set a distance with others who either take risks or are overcautious, inducing moral judgments associated with blaming and othering, aspects that I develop in Chap. 5.

The recurrent presence of emotions in prevention campaigns and official statements reveals that public health specialists maintain ambivalent relationships with emotions related to risk. A number of situations show that experts are not immune to emotional reactions themselves in the way they handle communication about health risks. Across various instances, they express fear but also contempt, disgust, or anger, as observed in smoking and obesity prevention campaigns: "Public health professionals also engage in judgments about risks and how best to deal with them that may be laden with intense emotion" (Lupton, 2013b, p. 642). These observations are aligned with the assumptions of moral panics, as a recurrent exaggeration of some situations defined as problematic, supported here by the moral judgments formulated by public health specialists and reinforced by the media.

Fear-based campaigns have been considered aggressive and paternalistic (Fairchild et al., 2018); however, they are sometimes presented as acceptable for reaching the ultimate goal of 'good health' through individual efforts. This confirms that the use of fear serves political interests (Gagnon et al., 2010) when considered a legitimate mode of governing a passive public. In parallel, other professionals who are in direct contact with the public in medical encounters, for example, feel like they have to perform 'emotion work': they strive to minimize anxiety when they balance the pros and cons of providing information about risks. These illustrations show the contradictions that exist between the limited place attributed to emotions in formal risk management and their role across a number of health risks. Their absence in this scholarship is associated with unawareness and misconceptions about the likelihood of panic or the legitimacy of using fear to convince. In that sense, emotions appear to have long been a *terra incognita* for decision makers. However, research on the topic is expanding and emphasizes the importance to address their role. Indeed, on the one hand, emotions obviously help to connect abstract risk knowledge and concrete experiences, but, on the other hand, they can be manipulative and counterproductive.

The fact that the value attributed to emotions is not symmetrical reflects power dynamics between experts and the public. On the one hand, emotions are seen as a source of bias when they are expressed in the public against the norms prescribed by public health institutions. On the other hand, they are perceived as legitimate resources for triggering changes when fear is purposively used in health education campaigns to alter social practices. Such asymmetry may more generally contribute to undermine trust in institutions. Using fear may backfire when, depending on how the threat actually materializes, the public questions official reactions manipulating evidence to either avoid overreactions or activate social responses.

In this chapter, I aimed to address the tension between formal risk management expectations to relieve fear through a reason-based approach to the future and the contemporary omnipresence of fear and anxiety. Illustrations have suggested that their presence should not be denied, including among professionals. Rather, it is critical to address emotions since they contribute to elaborate meanings and responses; therefore, they constitute an important dimension of health experiences. Challenging the cognitive framing of risk management, emotions bring into play bodily reactions, in addition to experiential knowledge, a combination of elements which help people to actually handle risk and uncertainty.

References

Armstrong, N., & Eborall, H. (2012). *The sociology of medical screening. Critical perspectives, new directions*. Wiley-Blackwell.

Bandes, S. A. (2008). Emotions, values, and the construction of risk. *University of Pennsylvania Law Review, 156*, 421–434.

Barbalet, J. (2002). Introduction: Why are emotions crucial. In J. Barbalet (Ed.), *Sociology and emotions* (The Sociological Review) (pp. 1–9). Blackwell Publishing.

Bauman, Z. (2006). *Liquid fear*. Polity.

Beck, U. (1992). *Risk society. Towards a new modernity*. Sage. [1986: first edition in German *Risikogesellschaft*].
Bericat, E. (2016). The sociology of emotions: Four decades of progress. *Current Sociology, 64*(3), 491–513. https://doi.org/10.1177/0011392115588355
Bombak, A. E. (2014). The "obesity epidemic": Evolving science, unchanging etiology: Unchanging etiology of obesity discourse. *Sociology Compass, 8*(5), 509–524. https://doi.org/10.1111/soc4.12153
Bonneux, L., & Van Damme, W. (2011). Health is more than influenza. *Bulletin of the World Health Organization, 89*, 539–540.
Bourke, J. (2006). *Fear: A cultural history* (1st ed.). Shoemaker Hoard: Distributed by Publishers Group West.
Bourrier, M. (2019). Comparing the 2009 A(H1N1) pandemic and 2014 Ebola virus disease. Of viruses, surprises in outbreak responses and global health work. In M. Bourrier, N. Brender, & C. Burton-Jeangros (Eds.), *Managing the global health response to epidemics: Social science perspectives* (pp. 73–104). Routledge.
Bourrier, M., Brender, N., & Burton-Jeangros, C. (Eds.). (2019). *Managing the global health response to epidemics: Social science perspectives*. Routledge.
Brodie, M., Brady, L. A., & Altman, D. E. (1998). Media coverage of managed care: Is there a negative bias? *Health Affairs, 17*(1), 9–25. https://doi.org/10.1377/hlthaff.17.1.9
Brookes, G., & Harvey, K. (2015). Peddling a semiotics of fear: A critical examination of scare tactics and commercial strategies in public health promotion. *Social Semiotics, 25*(1), 57–80. https://doi.org/10.1080/10350330.2014.988920
Bunton, R., Nettelton, S., & Burrows, R. (1995). *The sociology of health promotion. Critical analyses of consumption, lifestyle and risk*. Routledge.
Burton-Jeangros, C. (2004). *Cultures familiales du risque*. Economica.
Burton-Jeangros, C. (2011). Surveillance of risks in everyday life: The agency of pregnant women and its limitations. *Social Theory & Health, 9*(4), 419–436. https://doi.org/10.1057/sth.2011.15
Burton-Jeangros, C. (2019). Epidemics and risk communication. Why are lessons not learned? In M. Bourrier, N. Brender, & C. Burton-Jeangros (Eds.), *Managing the global health response to epidemics: Social science perspectives*. Routledge.
Burton-Jeangros, C., Aceti, M., Chappuis, P., Tsantoulis, P., & Hurst, S. (submitted). Bénéfices et limites de l'évaluation des risques de cancer par l'oncogénétique prédictive Une étude par forums citoyens. *Santé Publique*.
Burton-Jeangros, C., Cavalli, S., Gouilhers, S., & Hammer, R. (2013). Between tolerable uncertainty and unacceptable risks: How health professionals and

pregnant women think about the probabilities generated by prenatal screening. *Health, Risk & Society, 15*(2), 144–161. https://doi.org/10.1080/13698575.2013.771737

Burton-Jeangros, C., Fargnoli, V., & Petignat, P. (2015). To what extent will women accept HPV self-sampling for cervical cancer screening? A qualitative study conducted in Switzerland. *International Journal of Women's Health, 7*, 883. https://doi.org/10.2147/IJWH.S90772

Castel, R. (2003). *L'insécurité sociale: Qu'est-ce qu'être protégé?* Seuil.

Cavalli, S. (2014a). « Affiner le risque »: Les gynécologues-obstétriciens et la gestion des zones grises du dépistage de la trisomie 21. *Socio-anthropologie, 29*, 137–155. https://doi.org/10.4000/socio-anthropologie.1658

Cavalli, S. (2014b). *Gérer le risque et l'incertitude: Une typologie des stratégies professionnelles dans la pratique du dépistage prénatal* [Thèse de doctorat en sociologie, Université de Genève]. https://doi.org/10.13097/archive-ouverte/unige:40456

Chapman, G., & Coups, E. J. (2006). Emotions and preventive health behavior: Worry, regret and influenza vaccination. *Health Psychology, 25*(1), 82–99.

Clarke, L. (2002). Panic: Myth or reality? *Contexts, 1*, 21–26.

Clarke, L. (2006). *Worst cases. Terror and catastrophe in the popular imagination.* The University of Chicago Press.

Clarke, L., & Chess, C. (2008). Elites and panic: More to fear than fear itself. *Social Forces, 87*(2), 993.

Conti, K., Desai, S., Stawicki, S. P., & Papadimos, T. J. (2020). The evolving interplay between social media and international health security: A point of view. In S. P. Stawicki, M. S. Firstenberg, S. C. Galwankar, R. Izurieta, & T. Papadimos (Eds.), *Contemporary developments and perspectives in international health security.* IntechOpen. https://doi.org/10.5772/intechopen.93215

Davis, M., Stephenson, N., & Flowers, P. (2011). Compliant, complacent or panicked? Investigating the problematization of the Australian general public in pandemic influenza control. *Social Science & Medicine, 72*, 912–918.

Debergh, M. (2022). *La santé sexuelle à l'épreuve du local. Une ethnographie féministe en Suisse romande.* Université de Genève. https://doi.org/10.13097/archive-ouverte/unige:162733

Deml, M. J., Notter, J., Kliem, P., Buhl, A., Huber, B. M., Pfeiffer, C., Burton-Jeangros, C., & Tarr, P. E. (2019). "We treat humans, not herds!": A qualitative study of complementary and alternative medicine (CAM) providers' individualized approaches to vaccination in Switzerland. *Social Science & Medicine, 240*, 112556. https://doi.org/10.1016/j.socscimed.2019.112556

Doron, C.-O. (2009). Le principe de précaution: De l'environnement à la santé. *Les Cahiers du Centre Georges Canguilhem, 3*(1), 3–40. https://doi.org/10.3917/ccgc.003.0003
Earl, A., & Albarracín, D. (2007). Nature, decay, and spiraling of the effects of fear-inducing arguments and HIV counseling and testing: A meta-analysis of the short- and long-term outcomes of HIV-prevention interventions. *Health Psychology, 26*(4), 496–506. https://doi.org/10.1037/0278-6133.26.4.496
Ewald, F. (1996). *Philosophie de la précaution. L'Année sociologique, 46*(2), 383–412.
Fairchild, A. L., Bayer, R., & Colgrove, J. (2015). Risky business: New York city's experience with fear-based public health campaigns. *Health Affairs, 34*(5), 844–851. https://doi.org/10.1377/hlthaff.2014.1236
Fairchild, A. L., Bayer, R., Green, S. H., Colgrove, J., Kilgore, E., Sweeney, M., & Varma, J. K. (2018). The two faces of fear: A history of hard-hitting public health campaigns against tobacco and AIDS. *American Journal of Public Health, 108*(9), 1180–1186. https://doi.org/10.2105/AJPH.2018.304516
Fairchild, A. L., & Merritt Johns, D. (2015). Don't panic! The « excited and terrified » public mind from yellow fever to bioterrorism. In R. Peckham (Ed.), *Empires of panic: Epidemics and colonial anxieties* (pp. 155–179). Hong Kong University Press.
Fillion, E., & Torny, D. (2016). Un précédent manqué: Le Distilbène® et les perturbateurs endocriniens. Contribution à une sociologie de l'ignorance. *Sciences sociales et santé, 34*(3), 47–75.
Finucane, M., Slovic, P., Mertz, C., Flynn, J., & Satterfield, T. (2000). Gender, race and perceived risk: The « white male effect ». *Health, Risk & Society, 2*(2), 159–172.
Flint, S. W., Nobles, J., Gately, P., & Sahota, P. (2018). Weight stigma and discrimination: A call to the media. *The Lancet Diabetes & Endocrinology, 6*(3), 169–170. https://doi.org/10.1016/S2213-8587(18)30041-X
Francis, L. E. (2007). Emotions and health. In E. Stets Jan & H. Turner Joanthan (Eds.), *Handbook of the sociology of emotions* (pp. 591–610). Springer.
Freund, P. E. S. (1990). The expressive body: A common ground for the sociology of emotions and health and illness. *Sociology of Health and Illness, 12*(4), 452–477. https://doi.org/10.1111/1467-9566.ep11340419
Frey, B., Savage, D., & Torgler, B. (2010). Interaction of natural survival instincts and internalized social norms exploring the Titanic and Lusitania disasters. *Proceedings of the National Academy of Science, 107*(11), 4862–4865.
Furedi, F. (1998). *Culture of fear. Risk-taking and the morality of low expectation.* Cassell.

Gagnon, M., Jacob, J. D., & Holmes, D. (2010). Governing through (in)security: A critical analysis of a fear-based public health campaign. *Critical Public Health, 20*(2), 245–256.

Giddens, A. (1990). *The consequences of modernity*. Polity Press.

Giddens, A. (1991). *Modernity and self-identity in the late modern age*. Polity Press.

Gilman, S. L. (2010). Moral panics and pandemics. *The Lancet, 375*, 1865–1867.

Glass, T. A., & Schoch-Spana, M. (2002). Bioterrorism and the people: How to vaccinate a city against panic. *Clinical Infectious Diseases, 34*(2), 217–223. https://doi.org/10.2307/4461841

Glik, D. C. (2007). Risk communication for public health emergencies. *Annual Review of Public Health, 28*(1), 33–54. https://doi.org/10.1146/annurev.publhealth.28.021406.144123

Goode, E., & Ben-Yehuda, N. (1994). Moral panics: Culture, politics, and social construction. *Annual Review of Sociology, 20*, 149–171.

Gray, D. P., Dineen, M., & Sidaway-Lee, K. (2020). The worried well. *British Journal of General Practice, 70*(691), 84–85. https://doi.org/10.3399/bjgp20X708017

Guttman, N., & Salmon, C. T. (2004). Guilt, fear, stigma and knolwedge gaps: Ethical issues in public health communication interventions. *Bioethics, 18*(6), 531–552.

Guttman, N., & Lev, E. (2021). Ethical issues in COVID-19 communication to mitigate the pandemic: Dilemmas and practical implications. *Health Communication, 36*(1), 116–123. https://doi.org/10.1080/10410236.2020.1847439

Hammer, R. P., & Burton-Jeangros, C. (2013). Tensions around risks in pregnancy: A typology of women's experiences of surveillance medicine. *Social Science & Medicine, 93*, 55–63. https://doi.org/10.1016/j.socscimed.2013.05.033

Hammond, D., Fong, G. T., McDonald, P. W., Brown, K. S., & Cameron, R. (2004). Graphic Canadian cigarette warning labels and adverse outcomes: Evidence from Canadian smokers. *American Journal of Public Health, 94*(8), 1442–1445. https://doi.org/10.2105/ajph.94.8.1442

Hansson, A., Brodersen, J., Reventlow, S., & Pettersson, M. (2012). Opening Pandora's box: The experiences of having an asymptomatic aortic aneurysm under surveillance. *Health, Risk & Society, 14*(4), 341–359. https://doi.org/10.1080/13698575.2012.680953

Hastings, G., & Stead, M. (2004). Fear appeals in social marketing: Strategic and ethical reasons for concern. *Psychology and Marketing, 21*(11), 961–986.

Herzlich, C., & Pierret, J. (1989). The construction of a social phenomenon: AIDS in the French press. *Social Science & Medicine, 29*(11), 1235–1242. https://doi.org/10.1016/0277-9536(89)90062-2

Hill, D., Chapman, S., & Donovan, R. (1998). The return of scare tactics. *Tobacco Control, 7*(1), 5. https://doi.org/10.1136/tc.7.1.5

Hilton, S., & Hunt, K. (2010). UK newspapers' representations of the 2009-10 outbreak of swine flu: One health scare not over-hyped by the media? *Journal of Epidemiology and Community Health, 65*, 941–946.

Hochschild, A. R. (1979). Emotion work, feeling rules, and social structure. *American Journal of Sociology, 85*(3), 551–575.

Hughes, E., Kitzinger, J., & Murdock, G. (2006). The media and risk. In T. G. Peter & Z. Jens (Eds.), *Risk in social science* (pp. 250–270). Oxford University Press.

Ingraham, C., & Reeves, J. (2016). New media, new panics. *Critical Studies in Media Communication, 33*(5), 455–467. https://doi.org/10.1080/15295036.2016.1227863

Janis, I. L., & Feschbach, S. (1953). Effects of fear-arousing communications. *The Journal of Abnormal and Social Psychology, 48*(1), 78–92.

Johnson, N. R. (1987). Panic and the breakdown of social order: Popular myth, social theory, empirical evidence. *Sociological Focus, 20*(3), 171–183.

Kahan, D. M. (2008). Two conceptions of emotions in risk regulation. *University of Pennsylvania Law Review, 156*, 741–766.

Kasperson, R. E., et al. (1988). The social amplification of risk: A conceptual framework. *Risk Analysis, 8*, 177–197.

Kates, R. W., & Kasperson, J. X. (1983). Comparative risk analysis of technological hazards (A review). *Proceedings of the National Academy of Science, 80*, 7027–7038.

Kemper, T. D. (1991). Predicting emotions from social relations. *Social Psychology Quarterly, 54*(4), 330–342. https://doi.org/10.2307/2786845

Kilgo, D. K., Yoo, J., & Johnson, T. J. (2018). Spreading Ebola panic: Newspaper and social media coverage of the 2014 Ebola health crisis. *Health Communication, 34*, 1–7. https://doi.org/10.1080/10410236.2018.1437524

Kimber, L., Burton-Jeangros, C., Riom, L., & Hummel, C. (2018). Le sentiment d'insécurité chez les personnes âgées: Entre transformations de l'environnement et fragilité individuelle. *Swiss Journal of Sociology, 44*(1), 139–156.

Klemm, C., Das, E., & Hartmann, T. (2016). Swine flu and hype: A systematic review of media dramatization of the H1N1 influenza pandemic. *Journal of Risk Research, 19*(1), 1–20. https://doi.org/10.1080/13669877.2014.923029

Kok, G., Peters, G.-J. Y., Kessels, L. T. E., ten Hoor, G. A., & Ruiter, R. A. C. (2018). Ignoring theory and misinterpreting evidence: The false belief in fear appeals. *Health Psychology Review, 12*(2), 111–125. https://doi.org/10.1080/17437199.2017.1415767

Lakoff, A. (2017). *Unprepared: Global health in a time of emergency*. University of California Press.

Laurent-Simpson, A., & Lo, C. C. (2019). Risk society online: Zika virus, social media and distrust in the Centers for Disease Control and Prevention. *Sociology of Health & Illness, 41*(7), 1270–1288. https://doi.org/10.1111/1467-9566.12924

Lemal, M., & Van den Bulck, J. (2010). Television news coverage about cervical cancer: Impact on female viewers' vulnerability. *European Journal of Public Health, 21*(3), 381–386.

Lupton, D. (2013a). *Fat*. Routledge.

Lupton, D. (2013b). Risk and emotion: Towards an alternative theoretical perspective. *Health, Risk & Society, 15*(8), 634–647. https://doi.org/10.1080/13698575.2013.848847

Lutz, C., & White, G. M. (1986). The anthropology of emotions. *Annual Review of Anthropology, 15*, 405–436.

Mairal, G. (2011). The history and the narrative of risk in the media. *Health, Risk & Society, 13*(1), 65–79. https://doi.org/10.1080/13698575.2010.540313

Manaï, D., Burton-Jeangros, C., & Elger, B. S. (2010). *Risques et information dans le suivi de la grossesse*. Stämpfli.

Monaghan, L. F., Rich, E., & Bombak, A. E. (2019). Media, 'fat panic' and public pedagogy: Mapping contested terrain. *Sociology Compass, 13*(1), e12651. https://doi.org/10.1111/soc4.12651

Nerlich, B., & Halliday, C. (2007). Avian flu: The creation of expectations in the interplay between science and the media. *Sociology of Health & Illness, 29*(1), 46–65.

Norddal, G. A., Wifstad, Å., & Lian, O. S. (2022). 'It's like getting your car checked': The social construction of diabetes risk among participants in a population study. *Health, Risk & Society, 24*(3–4), 93–108. https://doi.org/10.1080/13698575.2022.2028742

Nussbaum, M. C. (2001). Emotions as judgments of value. In *Upheavals of thought: The intelligence of emotions* (pp. 19–88). Cambridge University Press. https://doi.org/10.1017/CBO9780511840715.002

Olin Lauritzen, S., & Sachs, L. (2001). Normality, risk and the future: Implicit communication of threat in health surveillance. *Sociology of Health & Illness, 23*(4), 497–516.

Oxman, A. D., Fretheim, A., Lewin, S., Flottorp, S., Glenton, C., Helleve, A., Vestrheim, D. F., Iversen, B. G., & Rosenbaum, S. E. (2022). Health communication in and out of public health emergencies: To persuade or to inform? *Health Research Policy and Systems, 20*(1), 28. https://doi.org/10.1186/s12961-022-00828-z

Patterson, M., & Johnston, J. (2012). Theorizing the obesity epidemic: Health crisis, moral panic and emerging hybrids. *Social Theory & Health, 10*, 265–291.

Peters, G.-J. Y., Ruiter, R. A. C., & Kok, G. (2013). Threatening communication: A critical re-analysis and a revised meta-analytic test of fear appeal theory. *Health Psychology Review, 7*(sup1), S8–S31. https://doi.org/10.1080/17437199.2012.703527

Powell, J. L., & Gilbert, T. (2008). Social theory and emotion: Sociological excursions. *International Journal of Sociology and Social Policy, 28*(9/10), 394–407. https://doi.org/10.1108/01443330810900220

Quarantelli, E. L. (1954). The nature and conditions of panic. *American Journal of Sociology, 60*(3), 267–275.

Quarantelli, E. L. (2001). The sociology of panic. In *International encyclopedia of the social and behavioral sciences*. Pergamon Press.

Rebughini, P. (2021). A sociology of anxiety: Western modern legacy and the Covid-19 outbreak. *International Sociology, 36*(4), 554–568. https://doi.org/10.1177/0268580921993325

Rose, G. A., Khaw, K.-T., & Marmot, M. G. (2008 [1992]). *Rose's strategy of preventive medicine: The complete original text* (New ed.). Oxford University Press.

Rossmann, C., Meyer, L., & Schulz, P. J. (2018). The mediated amplification of a crisis: Communicating the A/H1N1 pandemic in press releases and press coverage in Europe: The mediated amplification of a crisis. *Risk Analysis, 38*(2), 357–375. https://doi.org/10.1111/risa.12841

Saguy, A. C., & Riley, K. W. (2005). Weighing both sides: Morality, mortality, and framing contests over obesity. *Journal of Health Politics, Policy & Law, 30*(5), 869–921.

Schnittker, J. (2009). Mirage of health in the era of biomedicalization: Evaluating change in the threshold of illness, 1972-1996. *Social Forces, 87*(4), 2155–2182. https://doi.org/10.1353/sof.0.0218

Sheppard, B., Rubin, G. J., Wardman, J. K., & Wessely, S. (2006). Terrorism and dispelling the myth of a panic prone public. *Journal of Public Health Policy, 27*, 219–245.

Shilling, C. (2002). The two traditions in the sociology of emotions. In J. Barbalet (Ed.), *Sociology and emotions* (The Sociological Review) (pp. 10–32). Blackwell Publishing.

Slovic, P. (2000). *The perception of risk*. Earthscan.

Slovic, P., Finucane, M. L., Peters, E., & MacGregor, D. G. (2004). Risk as analysis and risk as feelings: Some thoughts about affect, reason, risk and rationality. *Risk Analysis, 24*(2), 311–322.

Starkstein, S. (2018). *A conceptual and therapeutic analysis of fear* (1st ed.). Springer International Publishing: Imprint: Palgrave Macmillan. https://doi.org/10.1007/978-3-319-78349-9

Stolow, J. A., Moses, L. M., Lederer, A. M., & Carter, R. (2020). How fear appeal approaches in COVID-19 Health communication may be harming the global community. *Health Education & Behavior, 47*(4), 531–535. https://doi.org/10.1177/1090198120935073

Sturdy, S. (2022). Framing utility: Regulatory reform and genetic tests in the USA, 1989–2000. *Social Science & Medicine, 304*, 112924. https://doi.org/10.1016/j.socscimed.2020.112924

Thoits, P. A. (1989). The sociology of emotions. *Annual Review of Sociology, 15*, 317–342.

Thomas, G. M., Roberts, J., & Griffiths, F. E. (2017). Ultrasound as a technology of reassurance? How pregnant women and health care professionals articulate ultrasound reassurance and its limitations. *Sociology of Health & Illness*. https://doi.org/10.1111/1467-9566.12554

Thompson, L. E., Barnett, J. R., & Pearce, J. R. (2009). Scared straight? Fear-appeal anti-smoking campaigns, risk, self-efficacy and addiction. *Health, Risk & Society, 11*(2), 181–196.

Turner, J. H., & Stets, J. E. (2006). Sociological theories of human emotions. *Annual Review of Sociology, 32*, 25–52.

Ungar, S. (1998). Hot crises and media reassurance: A comparison of emerging diseases and Ebola Zaire. *The British Journal of Sociology, 49*(1), 36–56. https://doi.org/10.2307/591262

Vasterman, P. L., & Ruigrok, N. (2013). Pandemic alarm in the Dutch media: Media coverage of the 2009 influenza A (H1N1) pandemic and the role of the expert sources. *European Journal of Communication, 28*(4), 436–453. https://doi.org/10.1177/0267323113486235

Walsh, J. P. (2020). Social media and moral panics: Assessing the effects of technological change on societal reaction. *International Journal of Cultural Studies, 23*(6), 840–859. https://doi.org/10.1177/1367877920912257

Warr, M. (2000). Fear of crime in the United States: Avenues for research and policy. In D. Duffee (Ed.), *Criminal justice 2000. Volume four: Measurement and analysis of crime and justice*. U.S. Department of Justice. National Institute of Justice.
Washer, P. (2010). *Emerging infectious diseases and society*. Palgrave Macmillan.
Wilkinson, I. (2001). *Anxiety in a risk society*. Routledge.
Williams, S. J., & Calnan, M. (1994). Perspectives on prevention: The views of general practitioners. *Sociology of Health and Illness, 16*(3), 372–393.
Witte, K., & Allen, M. (2000). A meta-analysis of fear appeals: Implications for effective public health campaigns. *Health Education and Behavior, 27*(5), 591–615.
Wynia, M. K. (2006). Risk and trust in public health: A cautionary tale. *American Journal of Bioethics, 6*(2), 3–6.
Zinn, J. (2006). Risk, affect and emotions. *Forum Qualitative Sozialforschung / Forum Qualitative Social Research, 7*(1), 29.
Zinn, J. O. (2016). 'In-between' and other reasonable ways to deal with risk and uncertainty: A review article. *Health, Risk & Society, 18*(7–8), 348–366. https://doi.org/10.1080/13698575.2016.1269879

4

Social Practices and Health Risks

Introduction

The idea of risk is tightly associated with actions to mitigate harm. Formal risk knowledge provides a blueprint for how institutions and individuals should behave across a number of domains to avert future harm. It sketches various scenarios that are more or less valued. This relates to a central question of sociology, that is, how much action is determined by the strength of social regulation and how much freedom individuals have amid collective expectations. It is quite obvious that, in any sociohistorical context, people do not act randomly: they are influenced by the social environment in which they live. Considering the current authority of science, rules formulated on risk evidence are expected by many to generate consensus and to lead to a unique set of actions, that is, people should avoid risk to maximize their self-interest. Nevertheless, individuals and communities regularly express their autonomy when they select which risks they want to avoid and which ones they are ready to take or ignore.

After the preceding chapters addressing how people know and feel about health risks, I discuss here how they actually act when confronted with future threats. The analysis of how recommendations formulated on

C. Burton-Jeangros, *Experiences of Health Risks*, Critical Studies in Risk and Uncertainty, https://doi.org/10.1007/978-3-031-65377-3_4

risk evidence are endorsed, or not, by individuals in their practices provides insights into the respective role of social structures and individual agency. I am particularly interested in the various arguments people use to justify either aligning their actions with public health recommendations or deviating from them. Formal risk management emphasizes the maximization of collective trade-offs between risk and safety, usually addressing risk issues in isolation and considering that this mechanism is similarly relevant for individuals' decisions. In social experiences, these views are contradicted by the prevalent value of individual autonomy, which, coupled with reflexivity prompted by access to multiple information, encourages more complex courses of action, potentially departing from those prescribed by institutions.

This contradiction is particularly true in the domain of health. Public health and medical advice regularly invites people to mitigate their personal risks while emphasizing personal responsibility in health decisions. In a top-down stance, experts frequently define members of the public as entrepreneurs of their own health, through a model of action in which they should systematically endorse risk-reducing strategies. However, across health risks, it is commonly observed that some people informed about potential harm make decisions that deviate from recommendations. Approaching these deviations as social practices set in their broader contexts helps understand the multiple forms of contestation that individuals develop against dominant norms. References to pleasure, moderation, a sense of personal immunity, and critiques of institutions explicitly challenge many risk management assumptions and reveal the complexity of risk experiences in society. This chapter presents a range of strategies and rationales underlying social practices related to health risks.

It starts with some insights into social action from a sociological perspective, followed by propositions of social theories of risk and sociology of health as regards social practices. I consider that these are helpful for better understanding the range of responses people adopt in front of prevention messages. In the second part, I illustrate these variations, with empirical findings across studies looking at people's motivations when they are faced with risk decisions.

Sociological Insights on Action, Risk, and Health

Sociological Models of Action

Sociological theory has formulated different models of action, endorsing various perspectives on the intersection between individuals and society. How much are individuals autonomous from external constraints and able to exert their free will to maximize their own benefits when selecting a certain course of action over various options? To what extent are their actions influenced by social structures and collective norms? Since this is not the place to provide a lengthy discussion about the multiple answers offered to these questions, I limit my presentation to a few elements that I consider useful for the analysis of social actions related to health risks described in the second part of this chapter.

Some sociologists focus on the agency of individuals who make decisions based on their motivations with the ultimate goal of maximizing their personal interest. Following approaches focused on purposive rational action, the 'homo economicus' model states that social order emanates from the sum of individual actions motivated by personal interest. An alternative view, initiated by Emile Durkheim, emphasizes the predominance of society over individuals, exerted through collective influences shaping individual actions. In this second model, labeled the 'homo sociologicus' model, social norms enforced through individual actions support social order (see, e.g., Reckwitz (2002)). Against this opposition, some authors have proposed theorizations reconciling the role of social structure and individual agency by considering that they inevitably interact in social practices (Bourdieu, 1979; Giddens, 1986). More recently, the theory of social practice, which offers a new perspective for approaching human behaviors, invites to tackle practices as bodily and mental activities integrating material objects, set in a background encompassing specific emotional and cognitive elements motivating action.

Three elements are worth mentioning in relation to developments in social practice theory. First, it encourages shifting attention to how people perform mundane and everyday actions. It thus stands against hyperintellectualization, which considers "human agency as a highly reflexive and formally rational enterprise which resembles to an amazing extent the self-images of modern intellectuals and their life-world – in the form of calculating or duty-obeying agents" (Reckwitz, 2002, p. 258). This has two important implications. On the one hand, concrete or material elements are important. The role of the human body in social action is emphasized: "A practice can be understood as the regular, skillful 'performance' of (human) bodies" (Reckwitz, 2002, p. 251). Beyond connecting mental or cognitive and bodily activities, it further invites paying attention to the role that objects play in social action, for example, a technology developed to support prevention (i.e., a vaccination). On the other hand, it stresses the routinized character of concrete contexts of actions. The fact that these are guided by a socially shared script and repeated across individuals facilitates everyday life and contributes to collective order through social reproduction. This means that unexpected circumstances and/or demands for changes in routines—such as those introduced by formal risk knowledge—are interrupting and questioning regular daily life, with discontinuities representing "crises of routines" (Reckwitz, 2002, p. 255).

Second, when sociologists consider the role of subjectivity or reflexivity in social action, they are interested in how agency may lead to practices that deviate from dominant social rules. Bourdieu (1979) elaborated this diversity in his detailed descriptions of variations in tastes across social positions, showing how routine actions are shaped by people's socialization. Giddens' (1991) emphasis on the reflexivity of social agents means that they navigate across multiple normative systems, suggesting that they are capable or even encouraged to act in ways that do not align with the script formulated by institutions. These approaches link the central role of cognitive and symbolic structures with the production of shared meanings to orient social action (Reckwitz, 2002). In these mechanisms, practices are shaped in interactions as a result of proximity to significant others and distance from distrusted others.

Third, actions are not static and do not occur as single or detached occurrences. Individuals are embedded in specific spatial and temporal contexts that impact their daily decisions. The dynamic nature of social practices is formulated in this statement about human agency as "a temporally embedded process of social engagement, informed by the past (in its habitual aspect) but also oriented toward the future (as a capacity to imagine alternative possibilities) and toward the present (as a capacity to contextualize past habits and future projects within the contingencies of the moment)" (Emirbayer & Mische, 1998, p. 964). Practices related to risk typically involve such a temporal dimension.

These theoretical insights are relevant for the upcoming discussion about social practices related to health risks since I consider important to situate actions in concrete social contexts, thus to encompass interactions and engagements with others. In addition, these insights question the capacity and willingness of individuals to change their behaviors in response to risk knowledge; indeed their health practices are organized as routines whose repetitive character facilitates social life.

Social Theories of Risk and Action

After revisiting various assumptions of risk management underlying official expectations toward action, I then move in this section to the contribution of the social theories of risk to the question of social action.

The blueprint for action suggested by formal risk management approaches is elaborated following the 'homo economicus' model of action, assuming that individuals behave with the intention to maximize their benefits over the costs of their actions. From this perspective, scientific evidence is expected to provide the knowledge necessary to define standards that are meaningful for all and lead to one single course of action. People's lack of adherence to risk recommendations has been attributed to faulty cognitive mechanisms biasing decisions (Slovic, 2000; Tversky & Kahneman, 1974). These initial but still influential assumptions have been challenged by the growing awareness of uncertainty, as I discussed in Chap. 2. The precautionary principle and possibilistic thinking, both questioning the relevance of risk probabilities, indeed encourage anticipatory action (Anderson, 2010). This means that the anticipation of a potentially adverse future is deemed sufficient to act in the present: "Common to all forms of anticipatory action is a seemingly paradoxical process whereby a future becomes cause and justification for some form of action in the here and now" (Anderson, 2010, p. 778). In that respect, precautionary and possibilistic thinking notably extend the scope of possible or desirable action to mitigate danger.

In addition to their focus on the globalization of risks, Beck and Giddens' writings also discuss the major consequences of risk for people's everyday lives. The obligation to choose among different "possible worlds" (Giddens, 1991, p. 29) means that individuals are regularly confronted with potentially difficult but engaging decisions. They are routinely asked to consider counterfactuals, with decisions that might later prove to be wrong. These demands do not sit comfortably with their need for a sense of ontological security, defined as "the confidence that most humans have in the continuity of their self-identity and the constancy of the surrounding social and material environments of action" (Giddens, 1990, p. 92). Douglas (1985) also emphasized the importance for individuals to define their self-immunity against the dangers of everyday community life, whose constant presence in society, through warnings in official and media channels, creates a sense of personal vulnerability.

Authors using Foucault's concept of discipline emphasized how formal risk knowledge gave power to institutions in defining appropriate action and organizing individual lives without surveillance being experienced as constraining: "advanced liberal rule seeks to govern through freedom, that is, through the regulated choices of individuals construed as autonomous and responsible subjects who live life as if it were an outcome of choice" (Sharon, 2015, p. 298). These scholars emphasize the subtle regulation of social practices and the reproduction of power relations between experts and members of the public through risk management. Following the initial focus on social control induced by risk surveillance, more recent work has, however, been interested in how people resist this normative context in some circumstances. It is thus proposed that the power exerted on people can be not only repressive and constraining, but also productive and enabling as already envisioned in Foucault's work (Sharon, 2015). These elements can be related to the interplay between structural determinants of action and individual agency.

By tackling the social acceptability of risk, Douglas (1985) pointed out the political character of decisions, and the possibility that people may respond to risk in different ways is entailed in her typology of four profiles defined at the intersection of two axes differentiating people's positions toward social structures and toward others (Douglas & Wildawsky, 1983). The grid axis considers people's relation to their social environment, as either tight or loose in regard to collective rules, and the group axis refers to social integration, as either individually focused or group oriented. She describes four ideal types of reactions to risk. Individualists are risk takers characterized by minimal social connections and avoidance of externally set regulations; bureaucrats are the opposite profile, being embedded in tight sets of relations and applying externally set regulations; egalitarians are socially integrated but reluctant to endorse outside regulations and thus claim alternative ways to act in front of danger; and the excluded group is little connected with others, while their actions are constrained by outside expectations, which means that they adopt a passive and fatalistic perspective on risks. This typology anticipates the coexistence of contrasted responses to risk situations, considering both individual agency and people's embedding in social structure and interactions.

The contribution of foundational authors to the social theories of risk mentioned in this section has mostly remained theoretical and has little engaged with empirical findings. This can be attributed to the difficulty of actually measuring risk-related social practices, which are much less often reported than 'risk perceptions'. However, how people rate risks does not necessarily align with their actions. In the second part of the chapter, I develop insights based on empirical research on health risks with the aim to better understand how individuals act in the face of future harm.

Sociology of Health Practices

Before turning to these empirical insights, I first present a number of theoretical elements developed in sociology of health. The importance attributed to individuals in the management of their health has radically changed over the past decades: in the mid-twentieth century, people were expected to visit doctors when they were sick, while today, they are repeatedly encouraged to promote their own health and anticipate risks in their everyday practices. In this section, I describe how they have been granted this agency in the shift from treating diseases to promoting their own health and acting early on pathological biomarkers, with a strong emphasis on their responsibility toward health. Then, I present various models of health behaviors proposed by health agencies, and recent developments in sociological theory about health practices are introduced.

Self-Responsibility and Autonomy Toward Health

In the founding work of medical sociology in the 1950s, Parsons (1951) proposed that medicine's role was to make sick individuals healthy again since their disease conditions were threatening the proper functioning of society. Without questioning the respective merits or limits of medicine, he portrayed passive individuals as happy to comply with medical recommendations. Although the legacy of his sociological perspective on medicine, then groundbreaking, should not be undermined, his propositions on the sick role have rapidly been challenged. The assumed compliance of sick individuals who would adhere to the prescriptions of doctors could only be maintained as long as medical power was uncontested. In the following decades, the adoption of an anthropological perspective 'at home'—that is, when scholars approached health and illness conceptions also in Western countries (Bury, 1997; Herzlich, 1992)—and the appreciation of patients' perspectives on their own illnesses emphasized their active role and likely conflicts with medical expectations (Freidson, 1988). In the context of chronic and long-term diseases, patients experiencing ailments over long periods of their life course became active players not only in their treatments but also in the prevention of risks. Currently, self-management models rely on the autonomy of patients who are considered able and willing to endorse some of the competencies previously attributed solely to professionals (Armstrong, 2014; Ménoret, 2015).

Within medicine, the emergence of bioethics also encouraged the increasingly active role of patients. The diffusion of informed consent procedures, incarnating the new normative imperative of individual autonomy in medical decisions (Corrigan, 2003), reflects a shift in power balance between providers and users of medical services. While the risks and benefits of medical procedures are constantly being weighed in clinical encounters, patients are nowadays regularly required to make personal decisions among a range of options, in circumstances in which uncertainty about the best course of action often prevails (Aronowitz, 2015).

In parallel to these important transformations within clinical settings, the surge of chronic diseases and the associated limits of medical responses gave new momentum to public health in the 1970s (Petersen & Lupton, 1996). Primary prevention campaigns promoted the self-responsibility of the general population toward health. The focus on lifestyles meant that members of the public would not only be expected to turn to professional help in case of poor health but also that they would pay continuing attention to their health in everyday life, representing an important extension of their duty toward their own health conditions. This extension was aligned with emerging conceptions equating personal responsibility with good citizenship (Crawford, 2006). It was also associated with expectations that members of the public endorsing autonomy would be eager to receive more information to guide their actions. At the same time, it implied an invasion of health concerns across their everyday private routines.

The success of health education over the past 50 years reflects the development of behavioral sciences, which are indeed very popular and continue to offer new insights into how to effectively modify social practices (e.g., Coreil, 2024). Primary prevention messages addressing the whole population a priori in good health aim at convincing people that they are actually vulnerable and capable of acting on risks. Some critics associate the emergence of individuals as 'health entrepreneurs' with larger transformations of the welfare state. Activation policies in the domain of unemployment are indeed aligned with public health focus on individual responsibility: "behaviorism has persisted as an approach in public health practice while simultaneously gaining credibility in other areas of public policy" (Crawshaw, 2012, p. 201). Such policies similarly stress that citizens are the agents of their own welfare and health. Encouragement to monitor one's health through constant self-tracking (with data on sleep, food intake, caloric burning, etc.) with connected devices can be seen as an extension of this general trend (Lupton, 2016).

In sociology of health, the limits of the health education model are regularly discussed. Marketing and communication strategies encouraging behavioral change still tend "to assume that people are blank sheets ready to be receptive to health promotion messages" (Baum & Fisher, 2014, p. 215). The legacy of these approaches is, for example, observed in obesity prevention: interventions remain focused on behavioral change despite growing evidence regarding the importance of broader social determinants (Blue et al., 2016; Fox et al., 2018). Despite the massive efforts in developing techniques for behavioral change, evidence of their efficacy remains limited (Cohn, 2014), and Meier states, "In reality, the beneficial effects of even well-designed information, education and social marketing interventions tend to be small, inconsistent and temporary" (Meier et al., 2018, p. 207).

In sum, reflecting medicine's growing uncertainty and declining power, people were increasingly granted responsibility for decisions related to their health. However, the constant extension of individual preoccupations with their health defined as a personal project has been questioned. It can be associated with the broader movement of biomedicalization encompassing everyday risk surveillance (Clarke et al., 2003). Conrad (1992) defined this focus on behaviors in everyday life as healthicization, in contrast to medicalization taking place in medical settings. Social scientists have also emphasized the shortcomings of the model of autonomy promoted by medicine and public health, since these disciplines assume that such autonomy leads to decisions and behaviors aligned with their recommendations.

In that respect, growing interest for health literacy among professionals reflects the expectation that the provision of adequate information may be sufficient to improve people's engagement with health institutions. However, it remains a top-down initiative that ignores the sociopolitical dimensions of literacy. In contrast, critical health literacy (Abel & Benkert, 2022) is an approach that acknowledges people's autonomy and empowerment toward the promotion of their own health through actions addressing the determinants of health inequalities, hence moving away from the individual focus of health education or health literacy models.

In other words, social scientists challenge the way responsibility and autonomy toward health are defined by health professions, considering that the latter often do not sufficiently consider the social embedding of health practices and risk decisions. I now move to forms of action developed in public health interventions that approach behavioral change with a different perspective on responses to health risks.

Additional Prevention Models of Actions

In addition to the main model of health education, various approaches to health risk prevention coexist within public health as a result of the variety of risks that professionals aim to prevent. Their specific features demand contrasted engagement of the general public or targeted categories. It is important to have these different models in mind, as well as the criticisms formulated by social scientists, since these approaches aim at providing guidance to people's daily practices, which are presented below.

Harm reduction strategies, developed in the domain of addiction interventions, pay attention to the adverse consequences of the promotion of abstinence or zero tolerance, notably in terms of moral judgments, since the practices continue to be used by some. The approach emerged in the 1960s and 1970s, promoted by activists (workers, doctors, programs, and policy-makers) opposed to drug use suppression and challenging the oppression of users (Roe, 2005). The HIV/AIDS epidemic generated additional support for this approach among policy-makers, seeing it as an opportunity to limit the transmission of the virus among people using drugs, hence limiting danger to wider society. What started as a 'bottom-up' process was then later 'mainstreamed' in some government policies. First adopted in Australia, the United Kingdom, Switzerland, the Netherlands, and Canada, it later extended to Asia, Latin America, and Central Eastern Europe (Ritter & Cameron, 2006). For example, the Australian government adopted a harm reduction strategy in alcohol prevention to develop "safer and healthy drinking cultures" (Keane, 2009), with a focus on three domains: road accidents, injury and violence, and social harms. In regards to smoking, considering that some individuals will continue smoking despite the identified adverse effects on their health (Choinière et al., 2007), priority was to be given to reducing the amount of smoking. Such modifications of the product itself have been supported by the tobacco industry since the 1950s through the production of cigarettes with filters, light cigarettes, or nicotine substitutes developed by the pharmaceutical industry since the 1980s. This model situates practices labeled as dangerous in their social environment, considering trade-offs between different types of harms, thus going beyond the individual focus of biomedical or epidemiological approaches.

In parallel, a number of public health crises, especially re-emerging infectious diseases, have challenged policy models based on risk evidence. Anticipating rare and incalculable events with massive consequences through possibilistic thinking in the aftermath of 9/11, governments initiated new strategies to engage the public in the management of collective health risks (Lakoff, 2017). The terminology of preparedness and readiness called for ongoing vigilance toward unexpected events. Preparedness is focused on the consequences of a crisis, since past occurrences showed that accidents or outbreaks cannot necessarily be averted by risk management. It requires the population to be on alert and ready to react rapidly in case of a public health emergency. The emphasis on people being constantly at risk, including facing unpredicted crises, "established the perfect machinery for placing the population in a constant state of readiness and awareness in regard their health" (Armstrong, 2014, p. 167).

The attention given to uncertainty and the precautionary principle also permeated a number of prevention campaigns addressing individual behaviors. The gap between evidence and prevention messages has been examined in debates about alcohol use during pregnancy (Schnegg, 2018). After campaigns warning women about the documented risks of smoking during pregnancy, alcohol consumption became a source of preoccupation. Health education materials produced in Scandinavian countries addressed the following question to pregnant women: "Why take chances?". Although evidence for the adverse consequences of moderate or low alcohol consumption is lacking, a large number of countries now advocate a total abstinence policy regarding alcohol consumption during pregnancy (Leppo et al., 2014). According to these authors, "the rationale for this ban whether or not it is explicitly stated is precaution, a response to uncertainty in which an outcome is considered so catastrophic that action is taken to mitigate it irrespective of probability of it occurring" (p. 524). Preemption strategies for potential threats have also been extended to smoking prevention in Australia (Diprose, 2008). Critics emphasize the paternalism of such public health strategies, which continue to extend the scope of anticipatory action in society.

In response to health risks, different forms of actions are thus prescribed by authorities through dedicated prevention campaigns and various forms of communication. Beyond health education, harm reduction strategies, preparedness, or precaution all try to engage the public in the reduction of multiple risks. Nevertheless, all these models of action share a central role attributed to individual responsibility, while they little engage with the heterogeneous social circumstances of the public.

From Health Behaviors to Social Practices Related to Health

In addition to critics addressing the behavioral change model, social practice theory (Reckwitz, 2002) is gaining credit in understanding people's reactions when faced with health risk information. In this section, I highlight the elements provided by this approach which help to situate action in its social contexts and amidst interactions.

Addressing the social embedding of practices leads to the expectation of the coexistence of contrasted health practices across the population, affected by cultural and structural variations. Such diversity exists against the dominant view of a unique course of action determined by the medical approach to health. In his elaboration of 'illness behaviors', Mechanic (1961) emphasized the limited overlap between social practices adopted in the face of illness and medical institution expectations. He pointed out the coexistence of multiple forms of action toward illness, including a large array of folk and lay forms of healing, indicating that a large amount of social practices take place outside of the medical environment. Decades later, Blaxter (2010) proposed this line of argument in the context of prevention. To reflect the recurrent gap between the medical behavioral model and actual prevention practices across the population, she coined the term 'enacted behaviors'. Interest in how individuals respond differently to prevention injunctions has also increased among scholars supporting the medicalization thesis. Initially, described as a top-down process, medicalization has increasingly been approached as an interactive process between professional and lay actors, with "a greater focus on the complex ways that people engage with the imperatives of healthy citizenship discourse" (Sharon, 2015, p. 298). Scholars have also noted that individuals often do not systematically either accept or reject healthy behaviors; rather, they may adopt discordant lifestyles. This reflects how health-related social practices interact in multiple, and possibly contradictory, ways with the rest of people's lives and their different social roles (Mollborn et al., 2021).

Health sociologists hence propose a shift of research toward social practices related to health, defined as "arrays of human activity which depend upon shared skills or practical understandings" (Meier et al., 2018, p. 208). Situating practices in their social context implies considering "the social, affective, material and interrelational features of human activity" (Cohn, 2014, p. 159). While the individualist model decontextualizes action, people are influenced by others and by social meanings attached to their social practices: "Health behaviors are not isolated individual decisions but embedded in people's deeply complicated social lives" (Mollborn et al., 2021, p. 399). Symbolic meanings and shared understandings attached to health-related action also relate to individuals' identity and position within society, as I further develop in Chap. 5. Their practices reveal and confirm their affiliations with and differences from others, according to the contrasted values they attach to health and other domains of life. Social practices theory also proposes paying attention to the material dimension of practices: promoting health requires specific materials or objects (healthy food, screening tests, vaccines). These require resources granting access to such material but also competencies and skills to be used (Blue et al., 2016). In addition, meanings are important in helping people connect with the materiality of these practices in their everyday life, making them either possible or not (Maller, 2015).

Another shift of perspective proposed by the theory of social practices is to consider practices rather than individuals: "the focus is upon practices, i.e., performances of routinized behaviors which are shared across groups of people" (Meier et al., 2018, p. 208). This means that a range of social practices often interact, such as alcohol use with other social practices entailing health risks (e.g. snacking) and occurring with other people. Therefore, it is important to consider 'bundles of practices'. Finally, the dynamic character of health practices is emphasized: "By studying how drinking practices fit with practices in other domains such as work, family and leisure, we can understand more clearly the processes of change and continuity" (Meier et al., 2018, p. 201). Many health practices—such as smoking, eating, using condoms, or respecting social distancing—take place in routine daily activities. These routine actions are concrete and continuous, and prevention messages calling for change may introduce a discontinuity, clashing with preferences for coherence and avoidance of conflicting practices (Blue et al., 2016). Indeed, both change and its absence must be justified toward others (family members, coworkers, etc.), who might prove supportive or resistant to change.

Additional insights into changes in practices related to health can be gained by using a life course perspective. The meanings and implications of specific health practices can greatly vary across life stages, while reflecting one's socialization, embodied social knowledge, and lived experiences (Savage et al., 2013). At the same time, transformations across historical time impacting successive generations are also important to consider (Mollborn et al., 2021). In her analysis of obese societies, Blue et al. (2021) indeed suggested that "seemingly private matters and individual problems [should be addressed] as sociohistorical issues" (p. 1054). The meanings and experiences attached to health issues vary depending on socioeconomic and environmental conditions. However, they also change as a result of developments in scientific knowledge and therapeutic solutions over time (e.g., with treatments for HIV/AIDS). Successive generations are exposed to these constantly changing conditions, creating potential tensions between cohorts.

In the next section, focused on health risks, I present empirical findings that describe the different responses people adopt when confronted with risks and the dilemmas these can raise. In a number of health domains, actions prescribed by health institutions are indeed met with a variety of responses, revealing people's agency and reflexivity through multiple forms of action.

(Re-)Actions Around Health Risks

I now mobilize qualitative studies on actions related to health risks to discuss the various arguments motivating practices related to health, in both their adherence to preventive norms and deviation from these expectations. The next sections describe practices related to health risks according to a continuum ranging between compliance, or even the extension of anticipatory action to encompass uncertainty, and resistance to risk reduction. The objective is to understand how people navigate across the multiple risk knowledges they are exposed to and how they use these to orient their everyday preventive actions.

From Self-Discipline to Anticipatory Action in the Absence of Evidence

Many people comply with formal risk prevention messages. This is regularly measured in quantitative population studies monitoring the proportion of people actually meeting official recommendations regarding eating habits, physical activity, use of alcohol and tobacco, and health screenings. Their motivations are rarely elaborated or problematized since they are consistent with professional expectations. However, it is still relevant to consider the rationale behind their actions. In that respect, insights into the trust people express toward official recommendations might be easier to capture in fateful moments, such as during pregnancy or genetic screening. Following tight risk monitoring, pregnant women have been observed to endorse individual responsibility consistent with medical recommendations with the explicit intention to minimize risks (Copelton, 2007). Some mothers reported being happy to delegate the surveillance of risks to experts: "I don't wonder much to be honest, for I trust medical staff to do the necessary tests [.] I fully trust the standards" (Hammer & Burton-Jeangros, 2013). This extended to practices in everyday life, with women valuing their capacity to avoid risks through the adoption of healthy lifestyles (Burton-Jeangros, 2011; Copelton, 2007).

The importance of healthy lifestyles is observed when people report that they endorse them in relation to some screening results, when these indicate, for example, that they present an elevated cholesterol risk or when men are informed that their prostate-specific antigen exceeds the average level (Gillespie, 2015). In our genetic cancer screening study, some participants associated being informed about an elevated risk of cancer with adopting healthier lifestyles to mitigate the risk of becoming sick (Burton-Jeangros et al., submitted). These findings show how much messages about healthy behaviors are largely disseminated as a legitimate response to a number of health threats. In addition to their role in primary prevention targeted to the general population, they have become 'preemptive therapies' in the context of secondary prevention (Gillespie, 2015).

The value of actions that protect against risks and alleviate fatalities has been publicly supported by Angelina Jolie's article in the New York Times on May 14, 2013, entitled 'My medical choice', in which she states, "I decided to be proactive and to minimize the risk as much I could. I decided to have a preventive double mastectomy". She acted before the onset of disease, based on probabilistic information. Such an imperative to act upon genetic information has been described in empirical studies, with women identified as being at elevated risk for breast cancer due to their genetic make-up emphasizing their agency: "I don't want to be a victim. I made a decision. I decided that… well, I'll block its [the gene's] path. I know that I carry the gene, OK, then I am not going to wait. No. Not this kind of fatalism. I will not end up like them [family members who died from cancer]. I'll live my own life" (Caiata-Zufferey et al., 2014, p. 4).

Compliance with recommendations might reflect a sort of blind trust in science and experts (Giddens, 1990), as well as in the set of guidelines they offer. Parents who comply with children's immunization schedule visit with pediatricians to follow the immunization standard protocol, as reported by this mother: "You can sense that it's organized (…) and that it's planned out, even for parents who have not yet accepted vaccination" (Deml et al., 2021, p. 46). Endorsing medical and public health advice is experienced as favorable, following the authority and regulation proposed by experts.

Regular risk surveillance has thus certainly gained an important place and is guiding social practices in multiple health domains. At the same time, its omnipresence and success induce further expectations for controlling undesirable outcomes. While experts started calling for anticipating incalculable risks, some members of the public now also worry about potential harm and adopt anticipatory action even in the absence of evidence. Under the tight medical and everyday life surveillance of risk during pregnancy, women are socialized into being constantly attentive to danger. It should therefore not come as a surprise when pregnant women and mothers worry about a number of risks they might impose on their (future) children, especially if experts advise for action even in the case of uncertainty, as in the case of alcohol consumption. In our study, pregnant women worried about the food they ate, as a potential vector of malformations, aware that such risks are small but also about other sources of danger, such as cosmetics, for the development of their fetus that are not yet documented. This supported the adoption of a precautionary position in everyday life, as formulated by this interviewee: "When in doubt, one does abstain from many things" (Burton-Jeangros, 2011, p. 426).

In their role as mothers, women have been privileged targets of medical supervision and prevention campaigns (Ehrenreich & English, 2005 [1978]). Their socialization into prevention means that they are inclined to adopt anticipatory action in the presence of uncertainty. Responses to the uncertainty surrounding the mad cow crisis at the end of the 1990s included anticipatory measures in a context of scientific uncertainty and in the absence of any official guidelines about beef consumption (Burton-Jeangros, 2004). A small proportion of the mothers who participated in that study reported having eliminated all the beef meat and related products to play it safe. This crisis can be considered an important milestone in the attention given to food in modern societies, with increasing awareness of the risks entailed by industrial food production. In more recent crises, ethnographic studies revealed how people exposed to the Chernobyl and Fukushima accidents struggled with the 'invisible' radio-nuclear risks whose existence has been denied by experts and authorities in both contexts (Kimura, 2016; Kuchinskaya, 2014). Maternal preoccupation with food in the aftermath of the Fukushima accident was raised in the absence of guidelines from authorities. Women claimed their agency by refusing to buy food from contaminated areas but also by attempting to establish their own evidence through the use of dosimeters to assess food nuclear contamination (Kimura, 2016). Hence, concrete strategies have been developed locally to address uncertainty.

These examples show how the different forms of thinking initiated by formal risk management are being integrated into a range of social practices aimed at protecting one's own and children's health. Ascertaining risks has more broadly fueled awareness of uncertainty across society. I suggest that the impulse to act in some circumstances despite the absence of evidence can be perceived as a form of agency, next to limited trust in medical recommendations and adherence to the precautionary principle. At the same time, anticipatory actions exponentially expand the domains of possible interventions, as well as areas of contention between groups of people interpreting risk and uncertainty in contrasting manners.

Pleasure in Daily Life Against Risk Prevention

In addition to responses seeking more control over the adverse health consequences of everyday life activities in the long run, I describe here other reactions focused on the immediate pleasure provided by a number of social practices qualified as dangerous by experts. They can be related to recent developments on the motivations and dynamics of risk-taking practices (Zinn, 2020).

A range of social activities encompass immediate enjoyable consequences for the self, in terms of pleasure associated with, for example, eating, smoking, drinking, or sexual interactions. The positive emotions associated with these actions conflict with risk prevention messages emphasizing the adoption of practices expected to avoid or delay the occurrence of diseases at a later stage in life (Coveney & Bunton, 2003). These risk-taking practices are often interpreted according to the concept of edgework coined by Lyng (1990), who suggested that some individuals learn to navigate between the gains associated with risk taking and the limits they still strive to respect to avoid chaos.

Empirical studies, while limited in number, have regularly pointed out how individuals, in some circumstances, prioritize immediate pleasure over discipline for long-term gains. In his description of two cultural accounts of health, Crawford (1984) described how some interviewees defined health foremost in terms of pleasure seeking, well-being, and enjoyment. To them, release was clearly preferable over a disciplinary regime promoted by health education, even though the latter might equate with better future health. A more recent study on the adoption of health lifestyles in Finland reported the presence of a pleasure repertoire in which interviewed individuals insisted on enjoyment as being part of a good life, whereas endorsing the dominant values of prevention could prove constraining (Pajari et al., 2006).

A similar balance between discipline and pleasure is reported in qualitative studies investigating the motivations of smokers: while they are aware of the dangers of their habits, they report that smoking is pleasurable and experienced as a relaxing habit (Katainen, 2006). Interpreted within their social circumstances, smoking offers a way to manage stress and dullness and provide affordable time off for those living in more deprived social circumstances (Peretti-Watel & Constance, 2009). In addition to these individual benefits, smoking also entails social relations with other smokers, which has positive consequences (Katainen, 2006). The social dimensions of binge drinking and eating have been explored in groups of hipsters and gamers (Cronin et al., 2014), emphasizing how these practices generated communities of consumption developing specific rituals of solidarity. The label of carnivalesque consumption underlines the temporary character of these extreme practices, allowing people to suspend the rules of ordinary life (Cronin et al., 2014): "In this way, the activity of edgework becomes a strategy to allow consumers to collectively rise above social demands, controls and regulations that attempt to dictate what's good or what's bad for individuals" (p. 1136).

These accounts confirm the importance of situating practices within their social contexts, since these shape individual actions sometimes against professional interpretative frameworks. Indeed, risk prevention often ignores the multiple ramifications of health practices in terms of identity and relations. People taking risks challenge the value of moderation, which gained a prominent place as an extension of the Protestant work ethic, emphasizing the importance of ascetism (Crawford, 1984). At the same time, some studies emphasize the presence of control, measured pleasure, or 'calculated hedonism' (Cronin et al., 2014). Hence, since risk-taking practices occur even when people are aware of the risks they expose themselves to, these findings suggest that some individuals might struggle to reconcile contradictory goals of their actions. Indeed, pleasure and hedonism have sometimes been acknowledged by prevention campaigns. In the context of HIV, some official messages from the early days of the epidemic associated safe sex and pleasure, departing from other campaigns emphasizing the control of risks through abstinence or stable relationships (Sandset et al., 2021). Health promotion messages in Danish campaigns have also acknowledged the importance of pleasure, adopting a less authoritarian view on health lifestyles (Karlsen & Villadsen, 2016).

According to the theory of social practices, these arguments related to concrete circumstances suggest that against the ascetic ethos promoted by risk evidence, some people place more value on the 'good life' rather than on the 'long life' underlying risk prevention (Sharon, 2015). A parallel can be made with the emergence of 'quality of life' in health care in the 1970s, in reaction to technological developments and medicalization striving to add years to life (Armstrong & Caldwell, 2004). Attention given to quality of life or well-being values people's immediate experiences rather than technical or medical quantitative gains. Such reasoning resonates with current concerns regarding sustainable development, which invites to value limitations over constant expansion.

A Sense of Low Personal Vulnerability

Another set of empirical results emphasizes the fact that people do not change their behaviors since they claim that they are less at risk than others; hence, social comparison processes are important. Across a number of contexts and issues, it has been observed that proximity to risks reduces salience and increases personal sense of control. Indeed, situations or settings defined as risky that have not brought any concrete adverse consequences yet encourage individuals to feel protected. Hence, past individual and collective experiences are likely to affect risk appreciations and influence practices. In this section, I discuss the arguments used by people to justify their distance from risk prevention as a result of their sense of personal immunity.

Quantitative studies have reported people's tendency to minimize or even deny personal health risks, while they acknowledge that these risks exist for others. These findings showed that across a range of threats, individuals rate their own risk of being affected as lower than that of others (Burton-Jeangros, 2004; Sjöberg, 2000). Research on infectious diseases confirms this phenomenon, in addition to observations made in the context of HIV/AIDS studies (Joffe, 1999), a systematic review of 2009 influenza a (H1N1) pandemic perceptions highlighted that most people considered themselves to be less at risk than others (Bults et al., 2015). Early results related to COVID-19 risk perceptions across four European countries (McColl et al., 2022) further confirmed this with individuals frequently stating that the risk for themselves was lower than that for others. Smokers often acknowledge that smoking is bad at the population level, but not for themselves specifically. By presenting smoking as a private active choice, they emphasize their self-control (Heikkinen et al., 2010). These attitudes tend to be associated with lower adoption of protective practices.

The literature on vaccine hesitancy is replete with illustrations of this mechanism. Mothers who are hesitant toward vaccines argue that their child is not the 'average child' targeted by immunization campaigns. They elaborate a symbolic border between their family and others valuing their own cognitive resources and supportive health practices, in comparison to others who are less fortunate (Senier, 2008). Claiming expertise as regard the specific needs of their own, unique, child, these mothers build what Reich (2014) calls an imagined 'gated community' protecting their children from dangerous outsiders, in association with their intense parenting habits. The idea of herd community promoted by authorities in charge of vaccination programs is therefore not relevant to them. This was explicitly formulated by complementary and alternative practitioners who commented on their interactions with parents about vaccination risks, as illustrated by the statement one of them formulated "We treat humans, not herds" (Deml et al., 2019). Hesitant or reluctant parents tackle vaccination as an individual choice, balanced against their other virtuous health practices, including diet, physical activity, sleep, and overall hygiene, that they consider sufficient to protect their family from infectious risks (Reich, 2020).

As further developed in Chap. 5, setting symbolic boundaries between the self and the dangerous 'other' or others at risk is a recurrent mechanism: it provides a possibility to feel safer and to claim agency over one's own practices, seen as protective in the context of a risk society which keeps stressing omnipresent threats to health. These boundaries illustrate the need for ontological security (Giddens, 1990) or subjective immunity (Douglas, 1985) evoked above, reflecting a fundamental hope that one is not constantly exposed to adverse risk situations, but rather can keep living with some sense of security. This separation of the self from others might be reinforced by the emphasis on self-responsibility toward health. Indeed, the promotion of autonomy—against the long-standing paternalism of health institutions—reinforces individuals' claims for self-regulation based on their personal appraisal of risks. Vaccine hesitancy more commonly observed among privileged families in affluent countries can thus also be interpreted as a form of social distinction (Bourdieu, 1979), emphasizing the endorsement of such personal responsibility. Indeed, identity work contributes to establish one's position compared to others (Mollborn et al., 2021).

These findings suggest that practices that do not mitigate health risks can be collectively defined as harmful, but as individually beneficial. Their adoption reflects the need to maintain a sense of personal immunity in everyday life, which contrasts with calls for being constantly alert to potential threats. This second position not only encourages a never-ending cycle of anticipatory action but also may contribute to the sense of vulnerability and prevalence of anxiety described in Chap. 3.

Private Choices Against Institutional Regulation

In a different line of argument, individuals justify their health practices in the larger environment in which these occur, emphasizing the detrimental role of external forces on individual health. In those accounts, individuals refuse to adopt practices prescribed by institutions because they do not trust these or consider them to be responsible for additional sources of risk. These justifications are often related to power relations.

Public health strategies aim at protecting population health while respecting individual freedom as a cardinal value in modern societies. Indeed, restrictions or calls for change in individual behaviors sometimes generate reactions against the 'nanny state' accused of paternalism (Calman, 2009). At the same time, it is acknowledged that in its duty to ensure conditions supportive of collective health, the state may have to restrict people's choices in some circumstances. Debates about potential COVID-19 vaccination mandates in 2021 reflected this tension between the state's duty to protect population health and individual autonomy.

It has been observed in the United Kingdom that organized groups of parents who voiced their concerns about vaccines, notably about the evidence of their benefits over their risks, encouraged other parents to become knowledgeable instead of blindly trusting official recommendations (Hobson-West, 2007). The efforts of providers to coerce parents into vaccinating their child, using fairly dramatic warnings about the consequences of the lack of immunization including threats that their child might die as a result of parental decision, may indeed contribute to parents' distrust (Deml et al., 2021). These top-down injunctions lead some parents to prefer complementary and alternative practitioners who take time to consider their concerns. Indeed, this study emphasizes that some parents explicitly question vaccination, as a result of their distrust toward biomedical providers who tried to persuade them to vaccinate their child. Vaccine hesitancy thus provides a good illustration of the tension between encouraging people to be entrepreneurs of their own and children's health and utilitarian public health advice (Reich, 2014).

In addition to claims for their individual autonomy over state regulation, some people question the independence of public institutions. Across a number of issues, including tobacco, H1N1, Zika, and COVID-19 vaccines, some members of the public express concerns regarding alleged conflicts of interest between public institutions and private industries (Laurent-Simpson & Lo, 2019; Peretti-Watel & Constance, 2009; Ward, 2023). They emphasize the hypocrisy of state institutions, which earn money through cigarette taxation; furthermore, they criticize the collusion between governments and various industries. The detrimental influences of the food and tobacco industry on policy-making have indeed been documented by researchers (Moodie et al., 2013; Sacks et al., 2018). These findings echo Douglas & Wildawsky's (1983) suggestion that those who are marginalized in society tend to not trust institutions and experts. Beyond alleged commercial influences, the reluctance of governments and agencies to question their past failures across various scandals, notably about vaccines in France and Italy (Attwell et al., 2022), is likely to further fuel mistrust toward institutions.

With these accounts, I aimed at presenting how various segments of the general public express serious critiques of risk management promoted by health institutions. As reflexive citizens accessing multiple sources of knowledge and reflecting on the shortcomings of risk evidence, they question the legitimacy of top-down strategies and shed light on the power relations taking place in the context of health risk regulation.

Trade-offs to Minimize Harm

Carried by the expectations of control of diseases and the associated zero-risk narrative, some prevention programs strive to eliminate risks. This is, for example, illustrated by the New Zealand program to be a smoke-free country by 2025. At the same time, more moderate approaches exist, such as harm reduction strategies, which illustrate efforts to consider exposing oneself to risk as acceptable through negotiations across different threats to health. The idea of harm reduction is in fact present in empirical studies of everyday life decisions. Individuals report practices aimed at establishing trade-offs between different adverse consequences through moderation and/or compensation across practices defined as dangerous, thus considering their practices in bundles as suggested by the theory of social practice. This could help to explain why discordant practices are commonly observed (Mollborn et al., 2021). In this section, I present qualitative findings documenting the negotiations people make to justify their unhealthy practices.

In everyday life, people commonly report their efforts to reduce harm through moderation strategies. Smokers mentioned limiting the number of cigarettes they smoke, such as setting a favorable comparison with those who were not able to establish such a personal limit and/or preferring light cigarettes (Heikkinen et al., 2010; Peretti-Watel &

Constance, 2009). Pregnant women who continue smoking describe their struggle to reduce smoking and to set some acceptable thresholds for themselves, as this woman proudly reported her success in limiting smoking while she was pregnant, reducing her consumption to half a cigarette and then to a third per day (Burton-Jeangros, 2011). Low-risk drinkers in the adult population also elaborate on their personal competence, which enables them to moderate their alcohol use through self-imposed rules regarding the number of drinks while being fully aware of the standards (Mugavin et al., 2023). Pregnant women described their personal negotiations as regard food labeled as risky while pregnant; they had reduced their intake of such foods without completely eliminating them (Burton-Jeangros, 2011): "Sometimes I ate salad when I should not have, well I was not totally obsessed by this" (p. 8). Others who were not fully compliant with norms considered that they were 'doing enough' (Copelton, 2007). These accounts reveal that people strive to control risks across situations by setting their own rules. If these do not match official rules, they still give them a sense of empowerment or agency based on their own standards.

These practices, which do not fully eliminate risks, are discussed in relation to their personal and social benefits. Alcohol enhances social interactions and is a personal reward in the context of daily life (Mugavin et al., 2023). The danger of smoking during pregnancy is balanced with the consequences of quitting, as reported by this interviewee: "I still smoke, and I've chosen to smoke two cigarettes per day in the evening because I enjoy it and I assume it's better to smoke them than bang my head against the wall" (Hammer & Inglin, 2014, p. 7). In all these contexts, interviewees are fully aware of the official norms and thus feel the necessity to justify their private arrangements with the rules. Furthermore, the moral pressure of risk guidelines is very present when pregnant women express the extreme guilt they feel by not being able to adhere to recommendations. Thus, they use some justifications to reduce cognitive dissonance, "stacking the facts", justifying their behavior (Wigginton & Lafrance, 2014, p. 537) during interviews. They provided indicators of the absence of harm to their children—"I am lucky they are ok"—while stating that smoking was beneficial to their own mental health. The participants appreciated the support of health professionals, whose authority made their deviation acceptable (Wigginton & Lafrance, 2014). This woman indeed indicated that her obstetrician had set an upper limit for her smoking: "He [obstetrician] told me that I could smoke up to five cigarettes, not more, and that I shouldn't get stressed out, that it shouldn't be a cause for anxiety" (Hammer & Inglin, 2014, p. 7). These accounts reveal the trade-offs performed across various consequences of risk practices, in this case balancing physical health risks to their children with their own mental health.

In summary, breaching public health norms regarding individual health prevention is common. People continue to endorse practices that entail some potential adverse consequences for their health; thus, they do not systematically respond to preventive action invitations. Resistance to dominant norms has been observed around all public health issues, ranging from risky lifestyles, vaccine hesitancy, or not up-to-date screening. At the same time, I showed that in many contexts people's accounts reveal the moral pressure associated with preventive expectations. Hence, I want to stress that they rarely simply adopt careless behaviors, rather they struggle with potential contradictions between their personal circumstances and dominant discourses (see Chap. 5).

Conclusion

The idea that health is doable, situated under the control of human agency, is recent. From this perspective, models of action promoted by health institutions emphasize the active role individuals should play in achieving good health across a large range of risks. They approach human action under the lens of homo economicus assumptions, considering that people who have appropriate information behave in ways that minimize the risks they are exposed to. However, I showed in this chapter that these assumptions oversimplify the complex nature of social practices.

The pervasiveness of messages about health risks means that today, all social practices potentially have an impact on health, and health-aware individuals are expected to pay attention to these consequences. However, studies show how these messages are met with multiple reactions, oscillating between overcompliance at one end, represented by practices influenced by precaution and uncertainty, and explicit resistance at the other end, with action that is not alleviating health risks as defined by experts. These practices rest upon contrasted relations with health institutions. Compliance and trust are present among those who prefer to delegate decisions to professionals, whose advice is then explicitly valued. However, other people are unsettled by the extent of potential danger, and their reflexivity questions the value and limitations of scientific evidence; their preoccupation and additional demands even create potential tensions with professionals. Still others express their lack of trust in institutions, motivated by skepticism toward the latter's performance and interrogations about the independence of official recommendations. As emphasized by Brown (2016), there exist complex relations between risk and trust that can both be used as coping strategies to face vulnerability.

This variety of social actions suggests that members of the public indeed validate the value of autonomy without simply endorsing the precepts of health institutions. Vaccine hesitancy nicely illustrates the contradiction between enforcing people's autonomy in health decisions, hence inviting them to opt out of vaccinations that are recommended and rarely mandatory, and the principle of solidarity underlying immunization programs. Hence, people express contrasting forms of proximity or distance from the abstract systems of science and medicine. In return, professionals feel more or less able and willing to respond to such variety of social responses.

In addition to formal risk management in the form of health education, strategies for harm reduction or precaution are also used in private health practices. Precautionary action suggests that anticipatory action even in the absence of evidence is sometimes deemed preferable. Following the motto 'better safe than sorry', safety should prevail over other considerations. However, the expectation to control any future potential harm may encourage overreactions when risk and uncertainty become performative despite being intangible entities. The emotional costs of these preventive actions should not be underestimated.

At the same time, findings suggest that people are rarely oblivious to formal risk injunctions and that those leaning toward harm reduction through moderation are aware of their lack of compliance. It can be associated with the expression of negative emotions, such as guilt and shame, as a result of not endorsing risk reduction. These emotional implications are not supportive of people's general health and well-being; their weight seems even greater among people taking responsibility for others, in care work, that is, most often women in charge of children and family health in general. Positions that explicitly question the legitimacy of health institutions in formulating risk recommendations may also have costs for those who hold them since their criticisms generate strong expert and public reactions that, at the end of the day, increase divisions in society, as I discuss in Chap. 5.

The theory of social practice helps to move away from the narrow behavioral focus of prevention campaigns. It considers how health practices are embedded in symbolic meanings and sets of values, such as the personal capacity for control over one's life conditions, projections toward the future, preference for delayed gratification over immediate pleasure, and health-related past experiences. All these affect the relevance of risk reduction messages. Material elements also matter in accessing health-promoting resources, such as access to food or leisure activities. Social practices related to health also depend on specific skills that individuals acquire and develop over time but that tend to be constantly questioned or revisited by new threats or changing official recommendations. In their everyday practices, people often have to arbitrate among various health behaviors that can compensate for each other. Contradictions and inconsistency indicate that these practices are not solely governed by the intention to maintain good health. Indeed, changes in practices advocated by formal risk knowledge disrupt routine social practices, which strive to leave adversity and uncertainty aside.

This chapter showed that the normative framework resting on formal risk management is regularly challenged in people's health experiences. This model, focused on cognitive processes of rational action, continues to be disseminated in campaigns emphasizing values of individual responsibility and self-realization around health (Mikkelsen, 2017) as an extension of activation policies attributed to neoliberal deregulation. However, it brackets out multiple aspects of social practices. In people's experiences, health often appears as something that is not just 'doable'. Health practices depend on their resources and social positions, as developed in Chap. 6. Furthermore, multiple external forces contradict individual efforts, be they genes, viruses, or industries. Health experiences thus suggest that the capacity for control promoted by prevention messages is not relevant and applicable for everyone.

References

Abel, T., & Benkert, R. (2022). Critical health literacy: Reflection and action for health. *Health Promotion International, 37*(4), 1–8. https://doi.org/10.1093/heapro/daac114

Anderson, B. (2010). Preemption, precaution, preparedness: Anticipatory action and future geographies. *Progress in Human Geography, 34*(6), 777–798. https://doi.org/10.1177/0309132510362600

Armstrong, D. (2014). Actors, patients and agency: A recent history. *Sociology of Health & Illness, 36*(2), 163–174. https://doi.org/10.1111/1467-9566.12100

Armstrong, D., & Caldwell, D. (2004). Origins of the concept of quality of life in health care: A rhetorical solution to a political problem. *Social Theory & Health, 2*(4), 361–371. https://doi.org/10.1057/palgrave.sth.8700038

Aronowitz, R. A. (2015). *Risky medicine: Our quest to cure fear and uncertainty*. The University of Chicago Press.

Attwell, K., Hannah, A., & Leask, J. (2022). COVID-19 : Talk of 'vaccine hesitancy' lets governments off the hook. *Nature, 602*(7898), 574–577. https://doi.org/10.1038/d41586-022-00495-8

Baum, F., & Fisher, M. (2014). Why behavioural health promotion endures despite its failure to reduce health inequities. *Sociology of Health & Illness, 36*(2), 213–225. https://doi.org/10.1111/1467-9566.12112

Blaxter, M. (2010). *Health* (2nd ed.). Polity.

Blue, S., Shove, E., Carmona, C., & Kelly, M. P. (2016). Theories of practice and public health: Understanding (un)healthy practices. *Critical Public Health, 26*(1), 36–50. https://doi.org/10.1080/09581596.2014.980396

Blue, S., Shove, E., & Kelly, M. P. (2021). Obese societies: Reconceptualising the challenge for public health. *Sociology of Health & Illness, 43*(4), 1051–1067. https://doi.org/10.1111/1467-9566.13275

Bourdieu, P. (1979). *La distinction: Critique sociale du jugement*. Éditions de Minuit.

Brown, P. (2016). Trust and risk. In A. Burgess, A. Alemanno, & J. Zinn (Eds.), *Routledge handbook of risk studies*. Routledge, Taylor & Francis Group.

Bults, M., Beaujean, D. J. M. A., Richardus, J. H., & Voeten, H. A. C. M. (2015). Perceptions and behavioral responses of the general public during the 2009 influenza A (H1N1) pandemic: A systematic review. *Disaster Medicine and Public Health Preparedness, 9*(2), 207–219. https://doi.org/10.1017/dmp.2014.160

Burton-Jeangros, C. (2004). *Cultures familiales du risque*. Economica.

Burton-Jeangros, C. (2011). Surveillance of risks in everyday life: The agency of pregnant women and its limitations. *Social Theory & Health, 9*(4), 419–436. https://doi.org/10.1057/sth.2011.15

Burton-Jeangros, C., Aceti, M., Chappuis, P., Tsantoulis, P., & Hurst, S. (submitted). Bénéfices et limites de l'évaluation des risques de cancer par l'oncogénétique prédictive Une étude par forums citoyens. *Santé Publique*.

Bury, M. (1997). *Health and illness in a changing society*. Routledge.

Caiata-Zufferey, M., Pagani, O., Cina, V., Membrez, V., Taborelli, M., Unger, S., Murphy, A., Monnerat, C., & Chappuis, P. O. (2014). Challenges in managing genetic cancer risk: A long-term qualitative study of unaffected women carrying BRCA1/BRCA2 mutations. *Genetics in Medicine, 17*, 726–732. https://doi.org/10.1038/gim.2014.183

Calman, K. (2009). Beyond the 'nanny state': Stewardship and public health. *Public Health, 123*(1), e6–e10. https://doi.org/10.1016/j.puhe.2008.10.025

Choinière, D., Rogers, B., & Kaiserman, M. J. (2007). Concepts liés à la réduction des méfaits dans la lutte au tabagisme. *Drogues, santé et société, 6*(1), 317–336.

Clarke, A. E., Mamo, L., Fishman, J. R., Shim, J. K., & Fosket, J. R. (2003). Biomedicalization: Technoscientific transformations of health, illness and US biomedicine. *American Sociological Review, 68*(2), 161–194.

Cohn, S. (2014). From health behaviours to health practices: An introduction. *Sociology of Health & Illness, 36*(2), 157–162. https://doi.org/10.1111/1467-9566.12140

Conrad, P. (1992). Medicalization and social control. *Annual Review of Sociology, 18*, 209–232.

Copelton, D. A. (2007). 'You are what you eat': Nutritional norms, maternal deviance, and neutralization of women's prenatal diets. *Deviant Behavior, 28*(5), 467–494.

Coreil, J. (Ed.). (2024). *Social and behavioral foundations of public health* (3rd ed.). Cognella.

Corrigan, O. (2003). Empty ethics: The problem with informed consent. *Sociology of Health & Illness, 25*(3), 768–792.

Coveney, J., & Bunton, R. (2003). In pursuit of the study of pleasure: Implications for health research and practice. *Health, 7*(2), 161–179.

Crawford, R. (1984). A cultural account of 'health': Control, release and the social body. In J. B. McKinlay (Ed.), *Issues in the political economy of health*. Tavistock.

Crawford, R. (2006). Health as a meaningful social practice. *Health, 10*(4), 401–420.

Crawshaw, P. (2012). Governing at a distance: Social marketing and the (bio) politics of responsibility. *Social Science & Medicine, 75*(1), 200–207. https://doi.org/10.1016/j.socscimed.2012.02.040

Cronin, J. M., McCarthy, M., & Collins, A. (2014). Creeping edgework: Carnivalesque consumption and the social experience of health risk. *Sociology of Health & Illness, 36*(8), 1125–1140. https://doi.org/10.1111/1467-9566.12155

Deml, M. J., Buhl, A., Huber, B. M., Burton-Jeangros, C., & Tarr, P. E. (2021). Trust, affect, and choice in parents' vaccination decision-making and health-care provider selection in Switzerland. *Sociology of Health & Illness, 44*, 41–58. https://doi.org/10.1111/1467-9566.13388

Deml, M. J., Notter, J., Kliem, P., Buhl, A., Huber, B. M., Pfeiffer, C., Burton-Jeangros, C., & Tarr, P. E. (2019). "We treat humans, not herds!": A qualitative study of complementary and alternative medicine (CAM) providers' individualized approaches to vaccination in Switzerland. *Social Science & Medicine, 240*, 112556. https://doi.org/10.1016/j.socscimed.2019.112556

Diprose, R. (2008). Biopolitical technologies of prevention. *Health Sociology Review, 17*(2), 141–150. https://doi.org/10.5172/hesr.451.17.2.141

Douglas, M. (1985). *Risk acceptability according to the social sciences*. Routledge & Kegan Paul.

Douglas, M., & Wildawsky, A. (1983). *Risk and culture: An essay on the selection of technological and environmental dangers*. University of California Press.

Ehrenreich, B., & English, D. (2005 [1978]). *For her own good. Two centuries of the experts' advice to women*. Anchor Books.

Emirbayer, M., & Mische, A. (1998). What is agency? *American Journal of Sociology, 103*(4), 962–1023.

Fox, N. J., Bissell, P., Peacock, M., & Blackburn, J. (2018). The micropolitics of obesity: Materialism, markets and food sovereignty. *Sociology, 52*(1), 111–127. https://doi.org/10.1177/0038038516647668

Freidson, E. (1988). *Profession of medicine: A study of the sociology of applied knowledge*. University of Chicago Press.

Giddens, A. (1986). *The constitution of society: Outline of the theory of structuration* (First paperback ed.). University of California Press.

Giddens, A. (1990). *The consequences of modernity*. Polity Press.

Giddens, A. (1991). *Modernity and self-identity in the late modern age*. Polity Press.
Gillespie, C. (2015). The risk experience: The social effects of health screening and the emergence of a proto-illness. *Sociology of Health & Illness, 37*(7), 973–987. https://doi.org/10.1111/1467-9566.12257
Hammer, R., & Inglin, S. (2014). 'I don't think it's risky, but…': Pregnant women's risk perceptions of maternal drinking and smoking. *Health, Risk & Society, 16*(1), 22–35. https://doi.org/10.1080/13698575.2013.863851
Hammer, R. P., & Burton-Jeangros, C. (2013). Tensions around risks in pregnancy: A typology of women's experiences of surveillance medicine. *Social Science & Medicine, 93*, 55–63. https://doi.org/10.1016/j.socscimed.2013.05.033
Heikkinen, H., Patja, K., & Jallinoja, P. (2010). Smokers' accounts on the health risks of smoking: Why is smoking not dangerous for me? *Social Science & Medicine, 71*(5), 877–883.
Herzlich, C. (1992). *Santé et maladie. Analyse d'une représentation sociale.* Editions de l'école des hautes études en sciences sociales.
Hobson-West, P. (2007). 'Trusting blindly can be the biggest risk of all': Organised resistance to childhood vaccination in the UK. *Sociology of Health & Illness, 29*(2), 198–215. https://doi.org/10.1111/j.1467-9566.2007.00544.x
Joffe, H. (1999). *Risk and « the other »*. Cambridge University Press.
Karlsen, M. P., & Villadsen, K. (2016). Health promotion, governmentality and the challenges of theorizing pleasure and desire. *Body & Society, 22*(3), 3–30. https://doi.org/10.1177/1357034X15616465
Katainen, A. (2006). Challenging the imperative of health? Smoking and justifications of risk-taking. *Critical Public Health, 16*(4), 295–305.
Keane, H. (2009). Intoxication, harm and pleasure: An analysis of the Australian National Alcohol Strategy. *Critical Public Health, 19*(2), 135–142.
Kimura, A. H. (2016). *Radiation brain moms and citizen scientists: The gender politics of food contamination after Fukushima.* Duke University Press.
Kuchinskaya, O. (2014). *The politics of invisibility: Public knowledge about radiation health effects after Chernobyl.* The MIT Press.
Lakoff, A. (2017). *Unprepared: Global health in a time of emergency.* University of California Press.
Laurent-Simpson, A., & Lo, C. C. (2019). Risk society online: Zika virus, social media and distrust in the Centers for Disease Control and Prevention. *Sociology of Health & Illness, 41*(7), 1270–1288. https://doi.org/10.1111/1467-9566.12924

Leppo, A., Hecksher, D., & Tryggvesson, K. (2014). 'Why take chances?' Advice on alcohol intake to pregnant and non-pregnant women in four Nordic countries. *Health, Risk & Society, 16*(6), 512–529. https://doi.org/10.1080/13698575.2014.957659

Lupton, D. (2016). *The quantified self: A sociology of sel-tracking*. Polity.

Lyng, S. (1990). Edgework: A social psychological analysis of voluntary risk taking. *American Journal of Sociology, 95*(4), 851–886. https://doi.org/10.2307/2780644

Maller, C. J. (2015). Understanding health through social practices: Performance and materiality in everyday life. *Sociology of Health & Illness, 37*(1), 52–66. https://doi.org/10.1111/1467-9566.12178

McColl, K., Debin, M., Souty, C., Guerrisi, C., Turbelin, C., Falchi, A., Bonmarin, I., Paolotti, D., Obi, C., Duggan, J., Moreno, Y., Wisniak, A., Flahault, A., Blanchon, T., Colizza, V., & Raude, J. (2022). Are people optimistically biased about the risk of COVID-19 infection? Lessons from the first wave of the pandemic in Europe. *International Journal of Environmental Research and Public Health, 19*(1), 436. https://doi.org/10.3390/ijerph19010436

Mechanic, D. (1961). The concept of illness behavior. *Journal of Chronic Diseases, 15*, 189–194.

Meier, P. S., Warde, A., & Holmes, J. (2018). All drinking is not equal: How a social practice theory lens could enhance public health research on alcohol and other health behaviours. *Addiction, 113*(2), 206–213. https://doi.org/10.1111/add.13895

Ménoret, M. (2015). La prescription d'autonomie en médecine. *Anthropologie et Santé, 10*. https://doi.org/10.4000/anthropologiesante.1665

Mikkelsen, H. H. (2017). Never too late for pleasure: Aging, neoliberalism, and the politics of potentiality in Denmark: Never too late for pleasure. *American Ethnologist, 44*(4), 646–656. https://doi.org/10.1111/amet.12563

Mollborn, S., Lawrence, E. M., & Saint Onge, J. M. (2021). Contributions and challenges in health lifestyles research. *Journal of Health and Social Behavior, 62*(3), 388–403. https://doi.org/10.1177/0022146521997813

Moodie, R., Stuckler, D., Monteiro, C., Sheron, N., Neal, B., Thamarangsi, T., Lincoln, P., & Casswell, S. (2013). Profits and pandemics: Prevention of harmful effects of tobacco, alcohol, and ultra-processed food and drink industries. *The Lancet, 381*(9867), 670–679. https://doi.org/10.1016/S0140-6736(12)62089-3

Mugavin, J., Room, R., Callinan, S., & MacLean, S. (2023). How do people drink alcohol at a low-risk level? *Health Sociology Review, 32*(3), 311–326. https://doi.org/10.1080/14461242.2023.2209090

Pajari, P. M., Jallinoja, P., & Absetz, P. (2006). Negotiation over self-control and activity: An analysis of balancing in the repertoires of Finnish healthy lifestyles. *Social Science & Medicine, 62*(10), 2601–2611. https://doi.org/10.1016/j.socscimed.2005.11.005

Parsons, T. (1951). *The social system*. The Free Press.

Peretti-Watel, P., & Constance, J. (2009). Comment les fumeurs pauvres justifient-ils leur pratique et jugent-ils la prévention? *Déviance et Société, 33*(2), 205–219.

Petersen, A., & Lupton, D. (1996). *The new public health. Health and self in the age of risk*. Sage.

Reckwitz, A. (2002). Toward a theory of social practices: A development in culturalist theorizing. *European Journal of Social Theory, 5*(2), 243–263. https://doi.org/10.1177/13684310222225432

Reich, J. A. (2014). Neoliberal mothering and vaccine refusal: Imagined gated communities and the privilege of choice. *Gender & Society, 28*(5), 679–704. https://doi.org/10.1177/0891243214532711

Reich, J. A. (2020). "We are fierce, independent thinkers and intelligent": Social capital and stigma management among mothers who refuse vaccines. *Social Science & Medicine, 257*, 112015. https://doi.org/10.1016/j.socscimed.2018.10.027

Ritter, A., & Cameron, J. (2006). A review of the efficacy and effectiveness of harm reduction strategies for alcohol, tobacco and illicit drugs. *Drug and Alcohol Review, 25*(6), 611–624. https://doi.org/10.1080/09595230600944529

Roe, G. (2005). Harm reduction as paradigm: Is better than bad good enough? The origins of harm reduction. *Critical Public Health, 15*(3), 243–250. https://doi.org/10.1080/09581590500372188

Sacks, G., Swinburn, B. A., Cameron, A. J., & Ruskin, G. (2018). How food companies influence evidence and opinion – straight from the horse's mouth. *Critical Public Health, 28*(2), 253–256. https://doi.org/10.1080/09581596.2017.1371844

Sandset, T., Villadsen, K., Heggen, K., & Engebretsen, E. (2021). Discipline for pleasure: A new governmentality of HIV prevention. *BioSocieties*. https://doi.org/10.1057/s41292-021-00257-1

Savage, M., Dumas, A., & Stuart, S. A. (2013). Fatalism and short-termism as cultural barriers to cardiac rehabilitation among underprivileged men. *Sociology of Health & Illness, 35*(8), 1211–1226. https://doi.org/10.1111/1467-9566.12040

Schnegg, C. (2018). *Éprouver le risque "alcool et grossesse" entre recherche, clinique et santé publique* [Thèse en sciences sociales, Université de Lausanne]. https://serval.unil.ch/resource/serval:BIB_1EB6CB5D3CDA.P001/REF.pdf
Senier, L. (2008). « It's your most precious thing »: Worst-case thinking, trust, and parental decision making about vaccinations. *Sociological Inquiry, 78*(2), 207–229.
Sharon, T. (2015). Healthy citizenship beyond autonomy and discipline: Tactical engagements with genetic testing. *BioSocieties, 10*(3), 295–316. https://doi.org/10.1057/biosoc.2014.29
Sjöberg, L. (2000). Factors in risk perception. *Risk Analysis, 20*(1), 1–12.
Slovic, P. (2000). *The perception of risk*. Earthscan.
Tversky, A., & Kahneman, D. (1974). Judgment under uncertainty: Heuristics and biases. *Science, 185*, 1124–1131.
Ward, J. K. (2023). Politisation et rapports ordinaires aux vaccins: Premiers enseignements de l'épidémie de Covid-19. *L'Année sociologique, 73*(2), 267–294. https://doi.org/10.3917/anso.232.0267
Wigginton, B., & Lafrance, M. N. (2014). 'I think he is immune to all the smoke I gave him': How women account for the harm of smoking during pregnancy. *Health, Risk & Society, 16*(6), 530–546. https://doi.org/10.1080/13698575.2014.951317
Zinn, J. (2020). *Understanding risk-taking*. Palgrave Macmillan.

5

Moral Judgments Around Experiences of Health Risks

Introduction

Risk is associated with collective and personal adverse events, hence it announces possible disruptions. As a result, it generates reactions toward maintaining social order. When dealing with risk, institutions and individuals elaborate different forms of social control: the distinction between proper and inadequate responses toward risks induces moral judgments. When they elaborate and disseminate such evaluations about the origin and management of disorder, people praise some individuals for their responses to risk while they devalue others. The latter is often the case for individuals or groups who do not act according to risk calculations; they are not only labeled but also blamed. These reactions stress the importance of social meanings constructed around risk, which form a normative framework. This normative framework is elaborated and maintained through social interactions, whether face-to-face or more frequently remote, based on faceless commitments in societies characterized by a high degree of specialization and division of labor (Giddens, 1990).

This chapter aims to address the mechanisms through which social norms are elaborated but also contested in relation to risk, next to

C. Burton-Jeangros, *Experiences of Health Risks*, Critical Studies in Risk and Uncertainty, https://doi.org/10.1007/978-3-031-65377-3_5

dynamic boundaries between safety and danger. On the one hand, the emphasis on human and individual responsibility in risk mitigation exacerbates the question of accountability: someone is to be blamed when risk is transformed into an adverse outcome. On the other hand, the multiple symbolic meanings that develop around new threats typically draw on preexisting divisions in society. Considering that risk surveillance introduces suspicion in social relationships, this chapter shows how interpretations of risk and uncertainty reinforce social and cultural divisions when making sense of emerging threats.

Preventive messages providing information on different health risks contribute to setting boundaries between others who are deemed dangerous—for example, because they are infected or because they smoke—and the virtuous self. Moral judgments associated with health risks typically use hierarchies defined by social differences, notably social class, race, and gender, and reproduce them. It is regularly observed that efforts to control risks generate othering and stigmatization toward those who adopt another appreciation of risk or integrate uncertainty in their evaluations. These social reactions are elaborated across various interpretations of risks, as formulated by scientists, policy-makers, media discourses, and everyday conversations. They have concrete implications for those who are blamed, as research shows that stigmatization and discrimination act as social determinants of health.

After introducing how sociological thinking addresses the permanent tension between individual autonomy and social order, I discuss the contribution of social theories of risk regarding the normative framework surrounding risks. I then present sociology of health insights about the role of moral judgments in shaping people's adoption of health advice and the consequences of stigma on the distribution of health. In the second part of the chapter, I summarize the empirical research on health risks to show how meanings actually reproduce social divisions while considering their diverse sources and consequences for risk surveillance.

The Normative Regulation of Risks and Health

Social Order, Social Norms, and Power Relations

The discipline of sociology developed at the end of the nineteenth century around emerging preoccupations in regard to the functioning of society. Emile Durkheim, one of the founding figures of the discipline, was foremost interested in understanding the capacity of social organizations to regulate themselves, managing to integrate individuals and social groups with diverging interests and preoccupations. Indeed, sociology, which then aimed to counter the economic perspective focused on the individual quest for self-interest, is particularly interested in how individuals incorporate the moral order of the society in which they live (Janowitz, 1975). The social fabric is maintained through norms, that is, assumptions shared by a number of individuals, which provide a common definition of situations, frame expectations toward others, and define specific ways to act in routine social circumstances (Ensminger & Knight, 1997). Fundamentally, social norms make social life possible by shaping interactions through the coordination of action across individuals. In other words, norms, which can be both formal and informal, organize mutual expectations and define common goals.

Living together is particularly challenging in times of social change. Durkheim was thus specifically interested in how social order could be maintained over the many transformations brought about by the industrial society, with needs for coordination between individuals and organizations at a larger scale than in previous centuries. At the end of the twentieth century, globalization brought again these questions to the fore at a broader scale, with concerns related to the management of global risk and uncertainty (Beck, 1992), as in the case of nuclear catastrophes or pandemics.

The interactions between the social organization and individuals, shaped by and reproducing social norms, define proper ways of living together. This implies different forms of sanctions directed toward individuals who do not respect norms. Indeed, conformity and social order are maintained as long as undesirable behaviors are identified and acted upon. These deviations have been examined under the lenses of deviance (Becker, 1997 [1963]) or stigma (Goffman, 1990 [1963]), which is of particular interest for the discussion of health risks below. For sociology, multiple definitions of deviance coexist, considering that it depends on how people react to each other's behaviors: "deviance is not a quality that lies in behavior itself, but in the interaction between the person who commits an act and those who respond to it" (Becker, 1997 [1963], p. 14). For Goffman, social norms define categories of ordinary action and deviant behaviors within specific interactional contexts. As a result of this categorization, social interactions are loaded with moral judgments toward others, whose behaviors are labeled either worthy or unworthy. Statements about what is safe and, by contrast, what is dangerous contribute to establishing such symbolic frontiers between valuable and depreciated responses—whether in meanings or in actions.

To achieve the overall goal of social order, moral judgments are associated with stigmatization toward people whose actions are not aligned with dominant norms. Indeed, stigma exists only through relations: "it should be seen that a language of relationships, not attribute is really needed" (Goffman, 1990 [1963], p. 13). Such relations, based on differentiated normative appreciations of others, reflect the distribution of power in society. Indeed, asymmetric relations facilitate stigma since it "it takes power to stigmatize" (Link & Phelan, 2001, p. 375). As developed later in this chapter, stigmatization occurring around health concerns is interlocked in contrasting ways with the power of officials associated with formal risk management in general and the medical profession in particular (Parker & Aggleton, 2003; Pescosolido & Martin, 2015).

These mechanisms geared toward sanctioning noncompliant individuals, potentially threatening social cohesion, consolidate the control exerted by those having power and their dominant position. Indeed, from a sociological point of view, such symbolic divisions are necessary since dominant positions can exist only against marginal positions. Beyond the lens of stigma, these enduring social processes have been approached through the concepts of blaming and othering. These emphasize the power imbalance that exists across social groups: "Othering is a practice that occurs when one group of people—usually a majority group or an in-group—treats another group of people—often a marginalized group or an out-group—as though there is something wrong with them" (Dionne & Turkmen, 2020, p. E214).

In the mid-twentieth century, scholars in deviance studies introduced an important contribution with their emphasis on how social norms shape interactions in power relations. However, they tended to approach those targeted by stigmatization as passive and unable to react against dominant norms (Anspach, 1979), even though Goffman (1990) considered their potential agency when discussing strategies of information management and the contingency of interactions. Since then, the capacity for resistance of those negatively labeled has been more and more considered, taking into consideration their potential for social mobilization against the moral judgments that keep depreciating them (Anspach, 1979).

Stigmatization and othering thus call for a theoretical approach addressing the relations or interactions generated by moral judgments. This requires further research beyond a focus on those suffering from stigma and their reactions to their spoiled identity. Indeed, attention must be paid to the 'moral entrepreneurs', defined by Becker (1997) as the people who actually define deviance. They are at the origin of labeling mechanisms and can induce discrimination, whether voluntarily or not (Scambler, 2009). This includes scientists and policy-makers, who produce social norms through risk communication, both in general and in the domain of health. Their messages encompass moral judgments and thus contribute to blaming, othering, and stigmatizing. The concept of 'stigma complex' (Pescosolido & Martin, 2015) aims at adopting such a broader perspective by paying attention to the transversal features of normative mechanisms that, across societies and multiple levels of analysis (from the biological to the social), transform differences into labels or marks that acquire social significance.

In summary, I presented different streams of research which have addressed issues related to the regulation of collective action through social norms shared in interactions. They concur regarding the recurrence of moral judgments in the maintenance of social order. Heterogeneous reactions toward danger generate judgments that either praise or alternatively devalue these reactions, in light of official recommendations. Through these processes, some categories gain or reinforce their standing, while others lose status. Below, I show that such power dynamics play out in the way health risks are addressed.

Social Theories of Risk and Social Order

The strength of technical risk management can be assessed through its capacity to set norms regarding proper versus improper responses to danger. Indeed, formal recommendations, largely circulated through official communication and media channels, set a normative framework that associates differentiated values with social practices adopted toward risks. Presenting some of these responses as inadequate or unworthy, by extension generates moral judgments toward those who adopt such responses.

Self Versus Others

As discussed in Chap. 4, new threats encourage individuals to reaffirm their own identity since danger jeopardizes their personal sense of security. Reaffirming social boundaries between the self and the rest of the world or, said differently, valuing one's in-group, reinforces a sense of low personal vulnerability. In addition, it prompts the formulation of shared understandings of risks that help to construct and strengthen a moral community whose members agree on the proper ways to deal with risk. This consensus produces cultural homogeneity within, in the sense of culture as "a system of persons holding one another mutually accountable" (Douglas, 1990, p. 10). At the same time, identity is elaborated and maintained through constant work of comparison with others (Joffe, 1999). This need for a sense of personal safety is encouraging to displace risks outside one's own group or community and, in return, it is fostered by the distance thus symbolically created with danger (Joffe, 1999). Blaming produces and maintains shared meanings within one's own group and consequently reinforces social cohesion in problematic situations. As formulated by Douglas (1995), the production of outsiders—through the ritual transfer of evil from inside toward the outside of the community—foremost serves to reinforce the order within.

The permanent search for a sense of personal safety encourages blaming and othering toward those who represent a potential source of disorder or chaos (Joffe, 1999). Agreements on how to handle danger reinforce lines of division toward others who do not think and act in the same way (Douglas, 1990). These differences are typically associated with preexisting social divisions and hierarchies. Social psychology refers to in-group and out-group, sociology to the division between 'them' and 'us', or 'insiders' versus 'outsiders'. These binary oppositions support existing representations of the world, typically shaped by power relations.

Douglas (1990) considers that increasing attention to risks—be they major or more mundane—contributes to mechanisms of stigmatization or blaming. Depending on their position in society, people react differently to new threats, endorsing the formal advice of authorities, or developing alternative narratives (see Chaps. 2 and 4). To defend their definition of the situation, those who are in a dominant position cast doubt and devalue those who do not adhere to their advice. In these processes, others are blamed to maintain social order. Douglas (1990) regrets what she termed 'the cultural innocence' of risk management and risk perceptions research, which has long ignored these persistent social processes: "there is nothing old-fashioned or exclusively primitive about social stereotyping. To assert that it is anomalous in our day is sheer cultural innocence" (pp. 14–15). From a socio-anthropological point of view, it is thus necessary to consider the situated understandings of danger that people elaborate when they are exposed to risks. The elements I presented thus far in this chapter help guide the discussion of empirical findings in the next section in two directions with, first, the role of moral entrepreneurs in blaming processes and, second, the capacity to resist of those who are blamed.

Risk Accountability: Who Is to Blame?

According to Giddens' (1990) statements about the disembedding of social relations, individuals are self-centered more than ever and less affiliated with others. This could mean that moral judgments formulated by others are less relevant; hence, people would be little affected by negative reactions generated by their own risk-taking practices. In parallel, formal risk management has profoundly expanded the focus on human accountability in relation to danger. According to the dominant narrative, accidents, catastrophes, or crises should have been averted (Bauman, 2006), and it is important to identify who is behind any harmful course of events. Efforts are thus made to associate a person with the unfolding from risks toward adverse outcomes, whether a fallible operator or the patient zero, for example. In contrast to other social environments in which causes of misfortunes are externalized to supernatural forces or gods' will (Alaszewski, 2015), the contemporary focus on human accountability has at least three consequences.

First, risk surveillance, supported by the constant reflexive monitoring of action (Giddens, 1990), contributes to the association of a single person or member of a group with the origin of a risk and its harmful unfolding. However, to be held accountable, people had to be informed about the risks. This explains why distance from knowledge might be preferable for some and ignorance may become 'strategic' (McGoey, 2012) to avoid being held accountable. Caduff (2014) associates the success of the precautionary approach with the increased accountability of collective and single actors who are summoned to subsequently justify the decisions they made in the past when an adverse outcome occurred later. To him, "precautionary action allows actors to leap over the gap that has opened up between the present moment of decision and the future moment of judgment" (p. 303). Hence, knowledge is not the sole driver of action and justification since moral judgments are anticipated in risk regulation.

Second, moral judgments and blaming can lead to formal sanctions. In his discussion of the crisis of responsibility generated by risk management, Giddens (1999) considers that the focus on human accountability reinforces litigation toward both officials and lay individuals. When misfortune is interpreted as the result of someone not properly averting risk, formal conviction can be warranted. This is, for example, illustrated by the legal actions taken against several scientists in the aftermath of the Aquila earthquake in Italy in 2009, who were accused of having underestimated the risks in information provided to the public a few days before the catastrophe. The criminalization of HIV-infected people who did not inform their sexual partners about their virologic status represents another form of litigation (Mykhalovskiy, 2011). These cases emphasize the individualization of responsibility and rest on a narrow understanding of the use of formal risk knowledge (see Chap. 2).

Third, the combination of elevated expectations for control and human accountability in case of adverse events encourages fear of human maleficence, as mentioned in Chap. 3. Against the suspicion that some individuals or groups might have evil motives toward others (Bauman, 2006), blaming and othering contribute to the attribution of accountability. These processes have consequences for social interactions in that they undermine trust in others. Thus risk management not only supports blaming mechanisms, but may more broadly contribute to weaken trust across society (Giddens, 1991).

To conclude this section on social studies of risk, I suggest that blaming associated with danger and misfortune is inherent to the way that risks are dealt with within social and cultural environments. The integration of risks possibly challenges the existing social order; thus it repeatedly produces symbolic interpretations, beyond risk knowledge, integrating moral judgments that situate individuals and groups in a normative landscape. Over time, the social acceptability of risks changes, creating tensions in interactions and changing patterns of blaming, yet they remain omnipresent.

Regulation of Health in Society

In regards to health, the institutions of medicine and public health have gained dominant positions in the management of disease and risk in modern western environments. They play a major role in the definition of how people should take care of their health, by formulating protocols for screening (cancer, hypertension, etc.), providing advice on everyday life behaviors (physical activity, eating, etc.), and preparing contingency plans in prevention of major public health events. The position occupied by these institutions is a result of their success in addressing diseases and in developing preventive strategies, but more broadly reflects the political process according to which other approaches to health and diseases (e.g., alternative medicine) have been devalued with the rise of modern medicine (Freidson, 1988). Accordingly, the diffusion of recommendations based on formal risk knowledge around health defines social norms: some forms of thinking and of acting are valued, while others are discarded. Professionals affiliated with medicine and public health act as 'moral entrepreneurs' (Becker, 1997). In other words, the rules and recommendations they formulate acquire moral connotations. I discuss here the implications of these moral judgments in two theoretical directions: first the concept of healthism emphasizes the moral value attached to good health, second stigmatization is approached as a social determinant of health, in interpersonal relations but also as a result of stigma conveyed amid social structures.

Prevention and the Moral Value of Health

As stated previously, the increasing capacity to accumulate and analyze data has extended the territory of health domains to act upon, in society and in the clinic (Armstrong, 2023). Indeed, in response to the identification of actionable risks threatening health—for example, an elevated risk of breast cancer as a result of genetic testing—more interventions—that is, a preventive mastectomy—are promoted. The pervasiveness of these norms has been criticized by scholars since the 1970s, according to their disciplinary power from Foucault's perspective (Petersen & Lupton, 1996), even though large segments of the public endorse public health and medical recommendations for risk reduction.

The extensive surveillance of health, over the whole lifespan from gestation to death, has generated a moral obligation toward being healthy. In affluent countries in which primary needs are met, the body and health have turned into symbolic sites of personal value, and they confer prestige to those who strive to preserve them. Crawford (1980) coined the term 'healthism' to emphasize the growing importance of health in society and the social control mechanisms associated with prevention. Against this background, individuals who do not make efforts toward their own health receive negative labels and are considered unworthy. Furthermore, the constant focus of risk factor epidemiology on individual accountability encourages the labeling of people in poor health since they are deemed responsible for their condition. Blaming the victim (Crawford, 1977) reflects still today a dominant narrative associating good health with individual efforts through healthy behaviors, while exonerating contextual determinants of health (see Chap. 6).

By defining what is 'normal', the normative framework of prevention shapes deviance. The role of health agencies in inducing stigma through prevention campaigns has been approached in various domains. In HIV/AIDS prevention, the potential discrimination of concerned people was emphasized early on, and in many contexts, it explicitly prompted messages countering the risk of stigma (Fairchild et al., 2018). In contrast, the denormalization of smoking, questioning a long-valued social practice, promoted efforts to control the tobacco epidemic, which attached stigma to smokers (David et al., 2024; Graham, 2012). Discussions about the ethics of using stigma in public health interventions, Bayer (2008) emphasizes the paternalism of prevention when it marginalizes the practices of some social groups. While some consider stigma to be a legitimate strategy to support healthy behaviors, others find it unacceptable or even a "barbaric form of social control" (Burris, 2008, p. 3). These insights show how much interpretations and actions related to health are deeply embedded in the social fabric.

Health Stigma as a Determinant of Health

As elaborated by Goffman (1990 [1963]) stigma is a social phenomenon that occurs in interactions and has consequences for people who are devalued. In recent years, health-related stigma research has expanded from an initial focus on mental health toward a number of conditions, notably HIV/AIDS or obesity (Pescosolido & Martin, 2015). Stigma means that "a difference is translated into a marked, devalued distinction" (p. 93). This difference is used to designate some persons as socially unworthy, and stigmatization refers to the process through which some individuals or groups in society attach stigma to others under specific health conditions.

These mechanisms have consequences: Hatzenbuehler et al. (2013) argue that stigma is a "driver of morbidity and mortality at a population level" (p. 813). It affects health status as an additional burden to individuals through the stress induced by adverse social reactions, impacting the resources available to them and their integration in society. Expanding beyond the role of stigma related to everyday social encounters, this research is interested in the role played by the social environment to address broader mechanisms: "Although widely acknowledged (but little studied), the role of context in shaping the lifestyles and life chances of individuals defines the nature of power and inequality, as well as normative determination of the good, the deserving, or the moral, and by contrast, the bad, the undeserving, and the immoral" (Pescosolido & Martin, 2015, p. 91).

According to formal risk management, adverse outcomes should be attributed to individual poor decisions, failure, or weakness. From a sociological perspective, they can be approached as the result of structural conditions that shape relations across different groups and produce social inequalities, as I further develop in Chap. 6. In this second reading, the understanding of stigmatization calls for a consideration of power relations in a specific social context that allow some groups to negatively label others, exposing them to additional adverse health consequences.

Social Regulation of Health Risks Through Othering and Blame

After the presentation of theoretical elements helping to understand the normative regulation of risks and health, in this second part of the chapter I bring together the historical, anthropological, and sociological literature addressing blame mechanisms related to various health risks, to discuss the content of these discourses, their different origins, and their consequences for concerned people and society more broadly. The identification and publicization of health risks have for a long time created new marks associated with prejudice and discrimination (Pescosolido & Martin, 2015). Such differentiated value can be related to bodies or biological conditions through marks that are visible on bodies (e.g., obesity) or in health practices (e.g., smoking) or to conditions not directly perceptible but open to suspicion (e.g., a person being a carrier of a virus).

Othering and Blaming Around Health Risks

Faced with the necessity of ensuring continuity and order in social activities, individuals have always elaborated responses to the occurrence of adverse events, as collective strategies to cope with danger and uncertainty. Social sciences disciplines (psychology, anthropology, sociology) use different terms to describe these mechanisms, including othering, blaming, stereotyping, scapegoating, or stigmatization. All these terms are loaded with moral judgments: they suggest that some people are deemed to be of less social value because of the health risks they are associated with.

Recurrent Lines of Social Division

Infectious diseases have been particularly prone to generate othering. Geographical borders are used to provide a sense of safety by attributing infections to those living elsewhere and by setting a physical frontier with them. When syphilis spread across Europe in the sixteenth century, its origins were located in the New World, while within Europe, it was systematically attributed to those living in another nation; for example, the Germans named it the French disease, while the French called it the Italian disease (Nelkin & Gilman, 1988). National borders have also been recurrently used in the context of re-emerging infectious diseases over the past decades. In the diffusion of HIV/AIDS, the blaming of people living in African countries, between France and the United States, or between the United States and Haïti has been common (Joffe, 1999). At the beginning of the twenty-first century, SARS and H5N1 were symbolically put at distance through discourses reinforcing the division running between the West and the East, with Asian countries blamed for their lack of preparedness and for not properly disclosing outbreaks (Washer, 2010). In the context of H1N1, narratives invoked the frontier between Mexico and the United States, and the rest of the world with negative reactions toward suspected carriers of the virus. The sense of protection associated with national borders was again made obvious in the early months of the COVID-19 pandemic when borders between countries were closed (Dionne & Turkmen, 2020).

The circulation of people through their migrant journeys provides another target for blaming. In the United States, Chinatown in New York and San Francisco have been historically portrayed as important reservoirs of infectious diseases (Dionne & Turkmen, 2020; Eichelberger, 2007), epitomized by the 1882 Chinese Exclusion Act. At the time of the SARS outbreak in 2003, Chinese migrants were again portrayed as a threat to the nation's health, morals, and technological superiority (Eichelberger, 2007). In the context of the COVID-19 pandemic, negative reactions toward migrants of Chinese or, more broadly, Asian origin have also been reported across multiple countries (Dionne & Turkmen, 2020; Labbé et al., 2022).

Divisions among religious affiliations are also commonly reported, with the circulation of religious communities seen as a source of danger. Jews were blamed for spreading the bubonic plague in the fourteenth century (Glick Schiller et al., 1994) and Muslims for the circulation of cholera in the nineteenth century during their pilgrimages to Mecca (Zylberman, 2007). In the context of the COVID-19 pandemic, Muslims in different regions of India were targets of blame and accused of spreading the virus (Dionne & Turkmen, 2020).

Dominant discourses typically use social distance to cast blame on those affected by infections. Over the course of the nineteenth century, cholera spread through industrialization, particularly affecting the poor concentrated in developing urban settings. They were blamed for their promiscuity, overcrowded housing, and alcohol use, all attached to immoral behaviors encouraging the spread of infectious diseases and more largely being a threat to the whole society (Nelkin & Gilman, 1988). In recent times, such divisions have focused on education rather than on social positions, with recurrent negative connotations toward people who do not adopt public health recommendations, hence not endorsing the model of behavioral change. In the context of COVID-19, the term "covidiot" was used in Canada to label those who refused to wear masks or get vaccinated, depicting them as silly and irrational (Labbé et al., 2022).

Social distance is further incarnated in danger associated with cultural practices that differ from those of people in dominant positions. In the early days of HIV/AIDS, based on emerging epidemiological knowledge, risks were associated with "people perceived as alien and exotic by scientists, physicians, journalists, and much of the US population" (Treichler, 1988, p. 42) due to their sexual or drug use behaviors. In the connections between HIV and Haïti, voodoo rituals were invoked. In the context of H1N1, SARS, and COVID-19, 'unsafe cultural practices' in regard to animals on Asian markets were noted. In Ebola outbreaks, local cultural practices—including funeral rituals and food practices (bushmeat consumption)—have been particularly blamed (Jones, 2011; Richards, 2016). In risk factor epidemiology, "culture itself is reconstituted as a 'risk factor' for infection in light of assumptions about African 'Otherness'" (Jones, 2011, p. 2). During the COVID-19 pandemic, episodes of hate crime toward people of Chinese origin exposed in the media supported the development of a general negative sentiment, leading to a broader devaluation of their cultural practices, deemed unsafe, as reflected in a disproportionate reduced attendance of Chinese restaurants, for example (Labbé et al., 2022).

Infectious diseases are particularly prone to raise moral judgments, as they potentially represent a threat for the whole society through their progressive diffusion across borders and social groups. Therefore, people who do not follow public health recommendations are sometimes labeled selfish. This has been observed in the case of resistance to official COVID-19 advice (Labbé et al., 2022), but more generally toward people who hesitate to vaccinate and thus do not contribute to collective safety (Attwell et al., 2022; Reich, 2020).

In primary prevention targeting smoking and eating habits, moral judgments are also frequent and often focused on 'insufficient education' or a lack of health literacy. Obesity and overweight generate negative social reactions, with fat people being blamed for their deviant bodies, not respecting the norms of control and moderation emphasized by modern public health regimes. These reactions encompass negative images of obese people, typically portrayed as greedy, lazy, or dirty (Lupton, 2013;

Saguy & Gruys, 2010). Moral judgments also concern parents of obese children blamed for not preventing overweight in their offspring; in particular, working mothers are frequently considered responsible for not inculcating proper eating habits to their children. Given that obesity is more prevalent among individuals in lower social classes, these opinions reflect and reinforce class divisions.

Long associated with social prestige, smoking status has changed over the course of a few years and is now associated with a range of negative attributes, with smokers qualified as dirty, addicted, selfish, stupid, and less productive at work (especially in the Anglo-Saxon world but also beyond) (Chapman & Freeman, 2008). The greater adoption of anti-smoking campaigns by more privileged social groups significantly altered the social distribution of smoking and, currently, negative attitudes toward smokers are indeed targeted toward less advantaged groups, blamed for their inability to change their practices (Graham, 2012).

These recurrent lines of division indicate that risk knowledge actually expands toward moral judgments: the social value of good health overlaps with the differentiated prestige of social positions. Some elements are worth highlighting across these regularities. First, blaming mechanisms are independent of formal risk knowledge. Uncertainty and the absence of evidence or experience can clearly exacerbate mechanisms of othering to restore a sense of self-immunity, as typically observed when new infectious diseases emerge, such as HIV in the early 1980s or COVID-19 in 2020. However, even when formal risk knowledge exists, moral judgments use social and political divisions that do not necessarily overlap with the actual distribution of a risk or a disease: "Associating a group with a viral pandemic does not have to be rooted in epidemiological data, as we recall how San Franciscans targeted the Chinese as a primary vector of infectious disease during the third bubonic plague, but did not subject Irish-born and other Caucasian immigrants to the same blaming and scapegoating, despite reports of a higher rate of infection among Irish immigrants" (Dionne & Turkmen, 2020, p. E223). In other words, sense-making and blaming align with political goals and are independent of actual health risks. This is further elaborated below.

Second, othering mechanisms according to geographical distance and social divisions are recurrent but dynamic. They adjust to the changing status of a health risk, its familiarity, and the moral judgments it generates, adapting to changing definitions of the social acceptability of different risks, such as smoking and obesity, which have in the past been associated with prestige. Nevertheless, the repetition of instances of blaming others in the context of disease is meaningful, confirming that defining the borders of safety and danger is an enduring social process. At the same time, these mechanisms keep reinforcing power positions over time. Geographical distance overlaps with long-established lines of devaluation formulated by Western countries toward those situated in the East and in the South. In addition, within countries, blaming groups according to preexisting lines of social classes or race and ethnicity reinforces the differentiated moral status of social categories. Indeed, blaming not only uses preexisting biases defined by sexism, racism, or classism, but also keeps reproducing them.

Third, blaming mechanisms should not be solely attributed to those in power positions. Their persistent character is illustrated by the way that those who are blamed and marginalized, in their turn, define 'others' who are dangerous, shifting their attention to less advantaged groups. In the context of SARS, long-settled residents in New York's Chinatown blamed more recent immigrants without a legal status and thus challenging the local labor market economy through accepting lower salaries (Eichelberger, 2007). Parents who do not vaccinate their children blame those who vaccinate without questioning the safety of immunization. To them, compliers are unhealthy; when endorsing official recommendations, they are described as sheep, lazy, and passive (Attwell & Smith, 2017; Reich, 2020). Therefore, some symmetry exists in blaming mechanisms: "the other 'forms' a potential repository of blame among hegemonic and non-hegemonic group members alike" (Joffe, 1999, p. 29).

In sum, I showed in this section that othering and blaming are persistent over time, circulate across society, and adapt to new threats. Moral judgments not only support a feeling of personal immunity but also help individuals face social disorder or restore social order, while maintaining their self-identity.

Sources of Blaming Mechanisms

In this section, I describe how the multiple origins of blaming narratives reinforce each other. Indeed, shared understandings emerge from the combination of enduring symbolic representations of illness in society, scientific theories, media, and political statements. They keep influencing each other and together produce a complex language around health risks.

Scientific Language and Health Communication

Scholars emphasize how the elaboration of scientific knowledge and its use in policy-making are shaped by social norms and reinforce them. Scientists play an important role in understanding diseases. While their statements are associated with scientific evidence, they contribute to blaming and othering strategies in their role as moral entrepreneurs.

In the nineteenth century, public health became very moralistic, sometimes referred to as "medical police" (Rosen, 1958), and presented disease as a penalty for immorality, with advocated measures targeting particular races and classes in the United States, including former slaves, immigrants, and religious communities (Bayer, 2008; Nelkin & Gilman, 1988). When HIV/AIDS emerged, the Centers for Disease Control and Prevention (CDC) in the United States defined epidemiological high-risk groups using geographical, social, and cultural categories to delineate safety and danger. The '4H' categories, pointing out homosexuals, hemophiliacs, heroin addicts, and Haitians, were defined to simplify complex transmission mechanisms into a few groups (Treichler, 1988). However, their emphasis on cultural practices, that is, sexual behaviors and drug use, which diverged from mainstream social practices, also served to establish a moral hierarchy (Glick Schiller et al., 1994). Treichler (1988) warned early on that "Ambiguity, homophobia, stereotyping, confusion, doublethink, them-versus-us, blame-the-victim, wishful thinking, none of these popular forms of semantic legerdemain about AIDS is absent from biomedical communication" (p. 37). The adverse impact of the dissemination of these shorthand labels in society was subsequently emphasized.

Public health has identified cultural practices as the source of health risks in other contexts. This was described in the lead poisoning 'epidemic' that developed into a public health concern in France at the end of the twentieth century (Fassin, 2005). More commonly observed among migrants, specialists attributed it to geophagy, an 'intentional' practice of eating earth by children, exposing them to lead paint flakes. This culturalist explanation was associated with Africans having migrated to France, emphasizing their 'exotic' social practices but without paying attention to their poor housing conditions, resulting from their precarious positions in the labor market, as the source of this outbreak. In Ebola-affected countries, public health professionals have also developed culturalist explanations focused on funerary rituals and eating bushmeat (Jones, 2011). Their calls for help from anthropologists reflect their hope that the latter's capacity to document cultural beliefs can provide tools to transform what specialists consider risky cultural practices.

The association between an emerging disease and the place and people it was first identified with is recurrent, as observed with SARS and China, H1N1 and Mexico, COVID-19 and China, and later variants in India and South Africa, both in popular but also in scientific language. Observing the adverse effects of the official naming of new diseases, the World Health Organization formulated a statement about best practices in 2015, recommending not using geographic location, people's names, animal or cultural references, or terms that amplify fear. These debates show the tension between labeling a new situation, which helps to formulate some understanding, and the social consequences of naming. They emphasize the inevitable intersection between science, policy, and society.

However, since the nineteenth century, health officials have also expressed preoccupation with the potential stigma attached to public health interventions. In the early days of the HIV epidemic, many public health professionals raised concerns about the potential for stigmatization of prevention campaigns. In France, Belgium, Switzerland, and the United States, campaigns were considered exemplary in that respect (Bayer, 2008; Pezeril, 2011). Attention to the risks of stigmatization and marginalization was also present at the international level within the World Health Organization and, later, the Joint United Nations

Programme on HIV/AIDS (UNAIDS), with a focus of communication and interventions on human rights and human dignity.

Indeed, prevention campaigns may have adverse implications for targeted populations. It has been observed that some tobacco control policies contribute to generating negative connotations associated with smokers, such as dirt and smell (Graham, 2012). Some scholars have therefore raised ethical concerns regarding the unintended or iatrogenic effects of 'hard-hitting' anti-smoking campaigns on smokers and people with lung cancer in terms of the stigma induced (Riley et al., 2017). The discussion is extended to the relevance of audience segmentation, which is sometimes adopted to improve the impact of campaigns. A systematic review emphasized the negative effects of health communication adopting this approach since communication specifically tackling ethnic and racial minorities using social comparison strategies—that is, emphasizing higher risks among some groups—reinforces the stigmatization of at-risk individuals (Peinado et al., 2020). Coupled with frequent individual responsibility framing, these messages support victim blaming, presenting those who are affected by a health issue (HIV, obesity) as weak or as lacking a sense of personal responsibility. The particularly strong impact in terms of stigmatization of visuals used in campaigns, compared to messages, has also been noted (Peinado et al., 2020).

With these elements, I suggest that in their activities and communication, scientists and public health specialists are not immune to blaming mechanisms, and these are likely to be quite largely disseminated as a result of the authority of science.

Politics and Policies

The movement of people across national borders particularly exacerbates anxiety related to epidemic risks. Over time, the overlap between health risk control and immigration concerns is shown through the regulation of people's circulation based on health grounds, with policies restricting travel or entry to people considered to present a threat (Bashford, 2006). The large increase in the number of pilgrims to Mecca in the late nineteenth century, at a time of increasing concern about infectious diseases in industrializing countries, led to the establishment of quarantine stations in Sinai in 1866, which imposed returning pilgrims to stop for 15 to 20 days when traveling on a boat with a suspected case of cholera (Zylberman, 2007). The United States practiced tight control at their borders in the late nineteenth and early twentieth centuries, refusing migrants with "loathsome or… dangerous contagious disease(s)" (in Fairchild & Tynan, 1994, p. 211), as well as in the Immigration Act of 1924, establishing restrictions based on eugenic arguments.

A century later, next to biosecurity concerns related to re-emerging infectious diseases, efforts to protect against dangerous others can be similarly observed. Such preoccupation developed in the United States in the aftermath of 9/11, associating disease control with military responses (Lakoff & Collier, 2008). It later permeated the World Health Organization, which dedicated its 2007 annual report to "*A safer future. Global public health security in the 21st century*" with an emblematic picture of the cover depicting a very dense a priori Asian city from a plane window. While attempts to quarantine HIV-infected individuals in the early 1980s were strongly criticized, the United States long denied entry to HIV-infected immigrants (Fairchild & Tynan, 1994). More recent outbreaks of infectious diseases, including H5N1, H1N1, Ebola, and COVID-19, have regularly reignited debates about border control strategies. Efforts to prevent the spread of viruses are at the same time constantly balanced against the economic impact of border closures. Indeed, with the revision of the International Health Regulation, enforced in 2005, the World Health Organization promotes the protection of public health while acknowledging "unnecessary interference with international traffic" (article 2), emphasizing the difficult connections between disease control and economic arguments. This debate became central during the successive waves of the COVID-19 pandemic, as the protection measures advocated by public health agencies were increasingly contested over time by those arguing for economic continuity.

Nevertheless, border closure as a strategy to protect against dangerous others was adopted by many countries in the early days of the first COVID-19 wave in spring 2020, in the absence of solid epidemiological evidence. While law scholars have debated whether border closure ran against the International Health Regulation, it is considered that it violated international human rights law (Chetail, 2020). This strategy certainly reinforced a sense of division between a safe space within the national territory against potentially dangerous others obliged to remain in other countries. Adverse reactions toward people of Chinese origin have been validated by politicians who vilified the role of China in the spread of the COVID-19 virus (Dionne & Turkmen, 2020). Ongoing controversies in the context of important geopolitical tensions, debates and uncertainty about the origin of the virus were thus used to reinforce political divisions (Dionne & Turkmen, 2020). This shows how much public health practices also contribute to conveying moral judgments toward others, depicted as either dangerous or safe, on the grounds of health risk control strategies.

Public health policies, sometimes coupled with migration policies, reinforce a normative framework that has consequences beyond health, with a detrimental impact on some groups of people. It turns out that they are more often those with less power in society (Graham, 2012). The role played by institutions and politicians in those mechanisms can be associated with structural stigma since their different forms of regulations restrict opportunities for some people (Pescosolido & Martin, 2015). In other words, I show here that both scientific and policy language have significant weight in society, and their role in the recurrence of blaming mechanisms should not be underestimated, especially in times of emerging threats.

The Media's Role in Othering Around Health Risks

Policy and scientific messages related to health risks are not only disseminated through official prevention campaigns and regulations, they are further circulated by the media. The latter play a central role in the integration of emerging diseases, but also of issues considered critical by public health, such as obesity and smoking, within society. Beyond providing an interface between scientists, experts, politicians, and the population at large (see Chaps. 2 and 3), I mobilize here research pointing out that the media contribute to divisions and blaming mechanisms.

In the early years of the HIV pandemic, coverage was low in the absence of a risk for the general heterosexual population. However, analyses have shown how AIDS initial media coverage reproduced dominant stereotypes, blaming homosexual men and people of African or Haitian origin in the spread of the epidemic (Sacks, 1996). As the virus circulation started to decline and treatments became available in the second half of the 1990s, media in the United States focused their attention on AIDS abroad. They then adopted an optimistic view about its control within the United States in contrast to the uncontrollable epidemic in African countries (Stevens & Hull, 2013). Blaming people in Africa for the continuation of the epidemic fed international public health preoccupations with the difficult control of infections in a globalized world.

Blaming can be conveyed in different ways. An analysis of images presented in the Swiss media in relation to H5N1 in 2005–2006 revealed the dichotomy suggested by the visuals between the Swiss technical control of infected poultry and the Asian lack of regulation and proximate relations between humans and animals in markets (Gorin et al., 2009). These images illustrate once again the symbolic distance established between another part of the world, Asia, which is depicted as outdated and unsafe, and the Western context, Switzerland, which is characterized by high protection standards. In the context of the COVID-19 pandemic and amidst the avalanche of media contents, a group of researchers have focused their attention on cartoons in the Canadian media, which are considered barometers of prevalent cultural attitudes and values (Labbé et al., 2022). Their analysis showed that these visuals reinforce moral judgments about the protection offered by political borders: foreigners, including people from China and from the United States, were presented as responsible for the spread of the virus; in addition, travelers and people living in cities compared to people in rural areas were portrayed as sources of danger.

Beyond infectious diseases, analysis of health risk coverage by the media repeatedly emphasizes the focus on individual responsibility (Saguy & Alemling, 2008). Messages about prevention thus not only reinforce the idea that individuals can control their health but also suggest that those who are not healthy lack a sense of personal responsibility.

This finding reinforces negative images associated with some groups of people, including those who smoke or those who are overweight.

These multiple forms of communication, combining official prevention campaigns, political positions, and media coverage of health risks, tend to reinforce each other and together feed everyday encounters in society, making othering mechanisms a normal part of the elaboration of meanings in the face of new health threats. These processes reflect the necessity of simplifying complex emerging situations presented as risky, which leads people, in their different social roles, to use preexisting or circulating categorizations when talking about these threats: "risk logics are shaped by symbolic systems expressed in various systems of classifications and taxonomies" (Alaszewski, 2015, p. 217). It is important to stress that scientific statements do not make symbolic responses redundant; rather, these continue to develop next to medical and statistical knowledge.

When these meanings associate social characteristics with different levels of risk, they both make use and reinforce the division of society into categories. As a starting point of many communication forms, epidemiology's potential for reinforcing racism, classism, sexism, or even placism (Smith-Morris, 2017) should thus be considered. Furthermore, scientific statements tend to have a long legacy in society, and original propositions might endure even when they become overridden by new scientific evidence. For example, while women treated for HIV are defined as having undetectable levels of HIV according to recent medical evidence, they are still exposed to discrimination, including from health professionals (Fargnoli, 2021). In other words, I consider important to take stock of the mutual influence of social, political, and media discourses that interact, feed, and reinforce each other, including their adverse consequences.

Consequences of Othering and Blaming

Beyond their role in elaborating collective meanings, blaming mechanisms have consequences for both the sources and the targets of these moral judgments. As discussed in Chap. 4, othering can contribute to complacency among those who convey it since the externalization of a health risk to other people can contribute to exposing oneself to risks (Dionne & Turkmen, 2020). For those who are blamed, othering can backfire through the explicit rejection of official statements. In other words, these mechanisms can run against public health recommendations rather than supporting them. In this section, I pay attention to the consequences of othering on interactions across groups, discussing strategies developed to cope with stigma and resistance toward official advice.

The Counterproductive Consequences of Stigmatization

The social processes discussed in this chapter emphasize how much interpretations and actions related to health are loaded with moral judgments: "Health and its meanings supply 'symbolic capital' for strategies of distinction and stigmatization" (Crawford, 2006, p. 403). These judgments toward those who represent a threat are spoiling their identity in Goffman's terms (1990 [1963]). Women who smoke during pregnancy report being exposed to social stigma and feel obliged to provide justifications of their behaviors to "repair" their negative identity (Wigginton & Lafrance, 2014). A systematic review emphasized how they experienced smoking during pregnancy as taboo and often felt "despised and disliked, and [...] perceived as irresponsible, selfish, or poorly educated" (David et al., 2024). Stigmatization emerges in actual interactions, for example, in the body language or comments of relatives of heterosexual women infected with HIV or in their encounters with health professionals (Fargnoli, 2021). However, it can also emanate from anticipated relations, leading to self-stigma, which reflects the incorporation by devalued people of the dominant negative representations of their condition: they endorse in advance the idea formulated by other people that they are less worthy (Pescosolido & Martin, 2015).

Alongside the distinction between a discredited and discreditable mark proposed by Goffman (1990 [1963]), people develop strategies to mask their association with a devalued condition or with a health risk. Some mothers who do not vaccinate their child report that in response to stigmatization, they avoid disclosing this information to reduce negative reactions (Reich, 2020). Women who smoke during pregnancy also avoid admission to their friends and relatives or in their encounters with health professionals (David et al., 2024). In Amoy Gardens in Hong Kong, a residential complex recorded with the world record of SARS cases (Lee et al., 2005), residents reported concealing their residential status when using services or applying for jobs. Such strategies, adopted to avoid blame, may reduce the social integration of those concealing their potential risks. Furthermore, it might exacerbate negative reactions toward them when they are discovered, leading them to remain even more entrenched in their views (Reich, 2020).

Thus, risk-related stigma has its own health consequences. It has been associated with deteriorated mental health among obese people (Puhl & Heuer, 2010). Widespread judgments about HIV-infected people may induce fear of social reactions whose consequences might be more detrimental than the actual infection itself, as stated by one HIV-infected heterosexual woman saying "she could die from the gaze of others" (Fargnoli, 2021, p. 215). These enduring social processes also limit the impact of prevention campaigns through a boomerang effect: messages emphasizing behavioral change are avoided or rejected by targeted audiences who do not want to be associated with negative images (Peinado et al., 2020). This may contribute to social and health inequalities across social groups. Individuals with a diminished status would not only take distance from advice, but also be particularly affected as a result of lower self-esteem, of fears associated with the uncovering of their condition in social interactions, and by the resulting social isolation. Consequently, prevention campaigns can in some circumstances contribute to the stigma described as a determinant of health (Hatzenbuehler et al., 2013).

These observations show the importance of considering how detrimental social interactions at the meso- and macrolevels interact with the poorer health of less advantaged groups in society. In that respect, the extent of stigmatization targeting women across a number of health risks can be related to the social control that public health and medical institutions, but also society at large, are exerting on their bodies, especially when they are deemed to expose others, their sexual partners, or their children, to undue risks (David et al., 2024; Fargnoli, 2021). This confirms that preexisting social divisions are reproduced in interpretations of health risks that circulate in society.

Resistance and Emancipation

In addition to research assessing the impact of stigma on devalued people's identity and health, this issue can be addressed through the lens of social resistance to dominant norms (Bayer, 2008; Scambler, 2009). Moving away from the image of passive recipients of stigmatization, the concept of 'identity politics' proposed by Anspach (1979) emphasizes the militant strategies elaborated by those labeled deviant. She defines identity politics as "a sort of phenomenological warfare, a struggle over the social meanings attached to attributes rather than an attempt to assimilate these attributes to the dominant meaning structure" (p. 773). Preexisting dominated positions according to characteristics that are devalued in the social environment, to which health risks are added, can end up in people endorsing a political role. Such a perspective has been observed in society and researched by the social sciences since the 1970s–1980s

Social and health mobilization occurred across a number of health-related domains, including HIV/AIDS, disability, obesity, and mental health. These movements are carried out by concerned people having a personal experience with these conditions, who sometimes have themselves an academic affiliation or are associated with researchers (Brown et al., 2004). Their mobilization aims at "transforming a personal trouble into a social problem" (p. 59) based on their personal experience while challenging medical and epidemiological narratives. This engagement reflects the capacity of some people to get together to denounce various forms of oppression, including from health institutions.

The HIV/AIDS epidemic revealed the potential for social mobilization against medical and public health perspectives. Homosexual men living in affluent countries intervened in the mainstream medical approach to the epidemic, managing to change scientific protocols and at the same time transforming societal views on homosexuality (Epstein, 1998). Their ability to do so was strongly supported by the economic, social, political, and symbolic resources of those among them who were occupying positions of power. In contrast, other highly affected groups, such as heterosexual women, are still struggling today to have their voices heard in dominant institutions (Fargnoli, 2021). As another illustration, mothers who are resistant to vaccination and who are often very active in searching for information and engaged in their parenting role use their social capital to develop networks and strategies to convince other parents not to vaccinate their children (Reich, 2020).

The capacity of some individuals to become active agents in their responses to health institutions is dependent upon their preexisting relations which can act as a motor of resistance: "We suggest that power relations within society, and the position of nondominant minority groups, may encourage members of these groups to actively engage, consciously or unconsciously, in different everyday resistance behaviors" (Factor et al., 2011, p. 1293). This resistance can remain implicit and individual based, or it can become collective and supported by peer groups. In the United States, the concept of 'acting white' has been proposed to suggest that some members of black minorities, as a result of their long-standing devalued status in society, deliberately reject behaving like the dominant group (Factor et al., 2011). These observations, that these authors propose to extend to other types of hierarchical social relations, emphasize the relational dimension of reactions to official recommendations.

In return, voices explicitly contesting the dominant narrative about health risks are currently addressed, from those in central positions, under the lens of conspiracy. It has been suggested that they can act as a 'rhetorical defense' (Farmer, 1992, p. 247) for groups who have little power in society. Such dissenting voices have long existed, already documented in the early days of vaccination campaigns at the end of the nineteenth century in the United States and the United Kingdom, with people expressing their distrust toward the government (Blume, 2006). Set in a global context, resistance to immunization observed in Pakistan is related to suspicions about the intentions of the state and might reflect the documented excesses of affluent countries strategies to eradicate smallpox (Kleinman, 2010). These campaigns, described as militarized and aggressive and conducted in the name of international public health interests, have indeed been shown to be disrespectful of local populations in that region (Greenough, 1995).

It is thus important to better understand the dynamics behind the formulation of conspiracy theories. Research suggests that the elaboration of these positions responds to three needs (K. M. Douglas et al., 2019): first, epistemic needs are prompted by curiosity and uncertainty avoidance; second, existential needs refer to the attempt to restore a sense of safety and control that has been weakened; and third, social needs relate to the importance of positioning oneself and one's group in a positive light. These elements suggest that conspiracy positions might in fact be reinforced by the relations prompted by blaming. These views are held by people fighting the dominant narrative that is shedding a negative light on them. In other words, the extent of conspiracy or social resistance might actually reveal the agency of those who are depreciated by the dominant narrative, which labels them as ignorant or idiot. In a relational perspective, blaming and othering should be considered symmetrical: those who are devalued formulate moral evaluations in return. Such resistance might further be fueled by feelings of injustice, which are present across various segments of the population.

In sum, I consider that blaming and the associated discrimination prompted by risk prevention interventions might contribute to impulse resistance, reflecting the capacity of reflexive publics to formulate critical positions toward health institutions and to elaborate claims for justice in their mobilization around health concerns.

Conclusion

Risk surveillance is embedded in social interactions that regulate reactions elaborated to face danger across society. This chapter shows that moral judgments around risk and uncertainty are common and develop along preexisting social and cultural divisions. Official risk messages unsettle the continuity of regular lives and consequently generate symbolic reactions. Therefore, risk regularly triggers mechanisms associated with "social categorization, division and cohesion" (Giritli Nygren et al., 2022, p. 111). Indeed, as discussed in Chap. 4, people strive to maintain a sense of self-immunity, which includes the aspiration to strengthen social cohesion with others who act similarly (Douglas, 1990). This implies reinforcing the distance from those associated with dangerous practices or attitudes. Findings presented in this chapter show that these divisions are systematic, observed over time and across sources of danger. They are elaborated across multiple sources of interpretations, including scientific statements, policy-making processes, media discourses, and everyday conversations. In these common social mechanisms helping to restore a sense of order and continuity, preexisting social categories offer ready-made lines of separation. The nowadays recurrent association of risk with human agency might even further reinforce such blaming of others, since the scientific narrative contributes to encourage the identification of the human source of misfortune.

Once it is established that othering and blaming are recurrent, it is important to consider their social implications. The adverse consequences of depreciation for those within society not adopting recommended behaviors, who are labeled uneducated, ignorant, or fatalist, should not be minimized. The authority of health professionals or politicians, who act as moral entrepreneurs, gives extra credit to these claims and thus exacerbates social hierarchies and the marginalization of less privileged categories. The reinforcement of social divisions generates stress, and stigmatization acts as a detrimental influence on personal health. It might additionally contribute to the radicalization of the positions of those who fight back, as a result of their adverse experiences of unfair treatment in the past.

The illustrations discussed in the chapter confirm the importance of considering actual experiences against the model of risk management. The cognitive framing of formal risk management is presented as an 'objective' approach to danger since it is based on numbers. As a result of the quantification of life, "We trust that numbers will be more transparent and objective than other forms of knowledge because we believe that numbers are impersonal; that the rules for producing them are clear, shared, and constraining; that their validity can be checked by others; and that their meanings are broadly interpretable" (Espeland & Vannebo, 2007, p. 38). However, the instances presented in the chapter challenge this vision since, in addition to quantitative figures, normative and political statements are constantly being formulated. In other words, science is socially embedded, and in their elaboration of risks and their interpretations, experts are regularly involved in mechanisms of blaming and othering.

Regulation through moral judgments pervades symbolic interpretations through interpersonal interactions but also through faceless commitments, prevention campaigns, or media contents. As health risks multiply, occasions of formulating moral judgments actually expand, including both calculated risks and conditions characterized by uncertainty as regard their potential for adverse outcomes. These judgments, fueled by the omnipresent attention given to health in modern societies, contribute to reshaping the moral fabric. Through blaming, othering, and stigmatization, biological vulnerability is transformed or expanded into social unworthiness when some groups are devalued by others. Such biosocial mechanisms are further addressed in Chap. 6. Indeed, the emphasis on individuals as the entrepreneurs of their own health contributes to blaming those who are in poor health, as it is attributed to their own responsibility while it neglects larger determinants of health.

Othering and stigma are situated within social hierarchies. While problematic others change over time, they always constantly only exist through relations that separate people into categories based on risks. Against the naturalization of health risks, the elements described in this chapter show that moral judgments beyond being present across society are also carried out by experts in different disciplines, as well as politicians, through their multiple forms of communication around health risks. Attention directed to the sources of othering and stigma has so far remained limited, this could be because it implies to question positions of power and privilege (Bayer, 2008). However, officials are moral entrepreneurs: they shape dominant narratives about emerging issues and frame issues in specific ways to gain collective attention. In that respect, Wailoo (2006) suggested that the prevention of risk represents a dilemma for public policy-making since the attention attributed to people who are more exposed can ultimately further reinforce their disadvantaged positions and negatively affect their health. In other words, power dynamics can reinforce the social and biological vulnerability of these groups through mechanisms of structural stigma (Pescosolido & Martin, 2015).

The attention given to health risks affects the way ordinary people think about their environment, behave, and relate with others through the informal regulation associated with moral judgments. Hence, othering and stigma around health risks have pervasive social consequences in terms of divisions. The repetition of these divisions across regions of the globe, as well as within countries across social categories, emphasizes their important social functions. At the same time, categories and divisions oversimplify complex mechanisms while encouraging the essentialization of groups or categories labeled as uniformly dangerous.

Against the emphasis on individual responsibility for health, I suggest in this chapter that variations in health status and health practices approached as individually preventable health risks contribute to challenge social cohesion. The language of risk can expand stigmatization since others are suspected of either not being sufficiently careful or in return to be too cautious. Finally, these considerations stress the tension that exists between the encouragement of autonomy and self-responsibility, on the one hand, and the value of solidarity, on the other hand, as regards health concerns in society.

References

Alaszewski, A. (2015). Anthropology and risk: Insights into uncertainty, danger and blame from other cultures – A review essay. *Health, Risk & Society, 17*(3–4), 205–225. https://doi.org/10.1080/13698575.2015.1070128

Anspach, R. R. (1979). From stigma to identity politics: Political activism among the physically disabled and former mental patients. *Social Science & Medicine. Part A: Medical Psychology & Medical Sociology, 13*, 765–773. https://doi.org/10.1016/0271-7123(79)90123-8

Armstrong, D. (2023). The social life of risk probabilities in medicine. *Social Science & Medicine, 323*, 115811. https://doi.org/10.1016/j.socscimed.2023.115811

Attwell, K., Hannah, A., & Leask, J. (2022). COVID-19: Talk of 'vaccine hesitancy' lets governments off the hook. *Nature, 602*(7898), 574–577. https://doi.org/10.1038/d41586-022-00495-8

Attwell, K., & Smith, D. T. (2017). Parenting as politics: Social identity theory and vaccine hesitant communities. *International Journal of Health Governance, 22*(3), 183–198. https://doi.org/10.1108/IJHG-03-2017-0008

Bashford, A. (Ed.). (2006). *Medicine at the border: Disease, globalization and security, 1850 to the present.* Palgrave Macmillan.

Bauman, Z. (2006). *Liquid fear.* Polity.

Bayer, R. (2008). Stigma and the ethics of public health: Not can we but should we. *Social Science & Medicine, 67*(3), 463–472. https://doi.org/10.1016/j.socscimed.2008.03.017

Beck, U. (1992). *Risk society. Towards a new modernity.* Sage. [1986: First edition in German *Risikogesellschaft*].

Becker, H. S. (1997). *Outsiders: Studies in the sociology of deviance* (New ed.). Free.

Blume, S. (2006). Anti-vaccination movements and their interpretations. *Social Science & Medicine, 62*, 628–642.

Brown, P., Zavetsoski, S., McCormick, S., Mayer, B., Rachel, M.-F., & Gasior Altman, R. (2004). Embodied health movements: New approaches to social movements in health. *Sociology of Health & Illness, 26*(1), 50–80.

Burris, S. (2008). Stigma, ethics and policy: A commentary on Bayer's "Stigma and the ethics of public health: Not can we but should we". *Stigma, Prejudice, Discrimination and Health, 67*(3), 473–475. https://doi.org/10.1016/j.socscimed.2008.03.020

Caduff, C. (2014). On the verge of death: Visions of biological vulnerability*. *Annual Review of Anthropology, 43*(1), 105–121. https://doi.org/10.1146/annurev-anthro-102313-030341

Chapman, S., & Freeman, B. (2008). Markers of the denormalisation of smoking and the tobacco industry. *Tobacco Control, 17*(1), 25–31. https://doi.org/10.1136/tc.2007.021386

Chetail, V. (2020). Crisis without borders: What does international law say about border closure in the context of Covid-19? *Frontiers in Political Science, 2*, 606307. https://doi.org/10.3389/fpos.2020.606307

Crawford, R. (1977). You are dangerous to your health: The ideology and politics of victim blaming. *International Journal of Health Services, 7*, 663–680.

Crawford, R. (1980). Healthism and the medicalization of everyday life. *International Journal of Health Services, 10*(3), 365–388.

Crawford, R. (2006). Health as a meaningful social practice. *Health, 10*(4), 401–420.

David, J.-C., Fonte, D., Sutter-Dallay, A.-L., Auriacombe, M., Serre, F., Rascle, N., & Loyal, D. (2024). The stigma of smoking among women: A systematic review. *Social Science & Medicine, 340*, 116491. https://doi.org/10.1016/j.socscimed.2023.116491

Dionne, K. Y., & Turkmen, F. F. (2020). The politics of pandemic othering: Putting COVID-19 in global and historical context. *International Organization, 74*(S1), E213–E230. https://doi.org/10.1017/S0020818320000405

Douglas, K. M., Uscinski, J. E., Sutton, R. M., Cichocka, A., Nefes, T., Ang, C. S., & Deravi, F. (2019). Understanding conspiracy theories. *Political Psychology, 40*(S1), 3–35. https://doi.org/10.1111/pops.12568

Douglas, M. (1990). Risk as a forensic resource. *Daedalus, 119*(4), 1–16.

Douglas, M. (1995). Risk and blame. In M. Douglas (Ed.), *Risk and blame. Essays in cultural theory* (pp. 3–21). Routledge.

Eichelberger, L. (2007). SARS and New York's Chinatown: The politics of risk and blame during an epidemic of fear. *Social Science & Medicine, 65*(6), 1284–1295.

Ensminger, J., & Knight, J. (1997). Changing social norms: Common property, bridewealth, and clan exogamy. *Current Anthropology, 38*(1), 1–24. https://doi.org/10.2307/2744433

Epstein, S. (1998). *Impure science: AIDS, activism, and the politics of knowledge* (Reprint). University of California Press.

Espeland, W. N., & Vannebo, B. I. (2007). Accountability, quantification, and law. *Annual Review of Law and Social Science, 3*(1), 21–43. https://doi.org/10.1146/annurev.lawsocsci.2.081805.105908

Factor, R., Kawachi, I., & Williams, D. R. (2011). Understanding high-risk behavior among non-dominant minorities: A social resistance framework. *Social Science & Medicine, 73*(9), 1292–1301. https://doi.org/10.1016/j.socscimed.2011.07.027

Fairchild, A. L., Bayer, R., Green, S. H., Colgrove, J., Kilgore, E., Sweeney, M., & Varma, J. K. (2018). The two faces of fear: A history of hard-hitting public health campaigns against tobacco and AIDS. *American Journal of Public Health, 108*(9), 1180–1186. https://doi.org/10.2105/AJPH.2018.304516

Fairchild, A. L., & Tynan, E. A. (1994). Policies of containment: Immigration in the era of AIDS. *American Journal of Public Healt, 84*(12), 2011–2022.

Fargnoli, V. (2021). *InVIHsibles: Trajectoires de femmes séropositives*. Editions Antipodes.

Farmer, P. (1992). *AIDS and accusation: Haiti and the geography of blame.* University of California Press.

Fassin, D. (2005). *Faire de la santé publique*. Ed. de l'École nationale de la santé publique.

Freidson, E. (1988). *Profession of medicine: A study of the sociology of applied knowledge* (University of Chicago Press ed.). University of Chicago Press.

Giddens, A. (1990). *The consequences of modernity*. Polity Press.

Giddens, A. (1991). *Modernity and self-identity in the late modern age*. Polity Press.

Giddens, A. (1999). Risk and responsibility. *The Modern Law Review, 62*(1), 1–10.

Giritli Nygren, K., Olofsson, A., & Öhman, S. (2022). Actor, structure and inequality: An intersectional perspective of risk. In D. Curran (Ed.), *Handbook on risk and inequality*. Edward Elgar Publishing.

Glick Schiller, N., Crystal, S., & Lewellen, D. (1994). Risky business: The cultural construction of AIDS risk groups. *Social Science and Medicine, 38*, 1337–1346.

Goffman, E. (1990). *Stigma: Notes on the management of spoiled identity*. Penguin.

Gorin, V., Dubied, A., & Burton-Jeangros, C. (2009). Une re-définition de la frontière Humain-Animal à travers les images des médias d'information suisses. *Studies in Communication Sciences, 9*(2), 191–220.

Graham, H. (2012). Smoking, stigma and social class. *Journal of Social Policy, 41*(1), 83–99. https://doi.org/10.1017/S004727941100033X

Greenough, P. (1995). Global immunizazion and culture: Compliance and resistance in large-scale public health campaigns. *Social Science and Medicine, 41*, 605–607.

Hatzenbuehler, M. L., Phelan, J. C., & Link, B. G. (2013). Stigma as a fundamental cause of population health inequalities. *American Journal of Public Healt, 103*(5), 813–821.

Janowitz, M. (1975). Sociological theory and social control. *American Journal of Sociology, 81*(1), 82–108. https://doi.org/10.2307/2777055

Joffe, H. (1999). *Risk and « the other »*. Cambridge University Press.

Jones, J. (2011). Ebola, emerging: The limitations of culturalist epidemiology. *Journal of Global Health, 1*(1), 1–5.

Kleinman, A. (2010). Four social theories for global health. *The Lancet, 375*(9725), 1518–1519. https://doi.org/10.1016/S0140-6736(10)60646-0

Labbé, F., Pelletier, C., Bettinger, J. A., Curran, J., Graham, J. E., Greyson, D., MacDonald, N. E., Meyer, S. B., Steenbeek, A., Xu, W., & Dubé, È. (2022). Stigma and blame related to COVID-19 pandemic: A case-study of editorial cartoons in Canada. *Social Science & Medicine, 296*, 114803. https://doi.org/10.1016/j.socscimed.2022.114803

Lakoff, A., & Collier, S. J. (Eds.). (2008). *Biosecurity interventions: Global health & security in question*. Columbia University Press.
Lee, S., Chan, L. Y. Y., Chau, A. M. Y., Kwok, K. P. S., & Kleinman, A. (2005). The experience of SARS-related stigma at Amoy Gardens. *Social Science & Medicine, 61*(9), 2038–2046.
Link, B. G., & Phelan, J. C. (2001). Conceptualizing stigma. *Annual Review of Sociology, 27*, 363–385.
Lupton, D. (2013). *Fat*. Routledge.
McGoey, L. (2012). Strategic unknowns: Towards a sociology of ignorance. *Economy and Society, 41*(1), 1–16.
Mykhalovskiy, E. (2011). The problem of « significant risk »: Exploring the public health impact of criminalizing HIV non-disclosure. *Social Science & Medicine, 73*(5), 668–675. https://doi.org/10.1016/j.socscimed.2011.06.051
Nelkin, D., & Gilman, S. L. (1988). Placing blame for devastating disease. *Social Research, 55*(3), 361–378.
Parker, R., & Aggleton, P. (2003). HIV and AIDS-related stigma and discrimination: A conceptual framework and implications for action. *Social Science & Medicine, 57*, 13–24.
Peinado, S., Treiman, K., Uhrig, J. D., Taylor, J. C., & Stryker, J. E. (2020). Effectively communicating about HIV and other health disparities: Findings from a literature review and future directions. *Frontiers in Communication, 5*, 539174. https://doi.org/10.3389/fcomm.2020.539174
Pescosolido, B. A., & Martin, J. K. (2015). The stigma complex. *Annual Review of Sociology, 41*(1), 87–116. https://doi.org/10.1146/annurev-soc-071312-145702
Petersen, A., & Lupton, D. (1996). *The new public health. Health and self in the age of risk*. Sage.
Pezeril, C. (2011). Le dégoût dans les campagnes de lutte contre le sida. *Ethnologie française, 41*(1), 79–88. https://doi.org/10.3917/ethn.111.0079
Puhl, R. M., & Heuer, C. A. (2010). Obesity stigma: Important considerations for public health. *American Journal of Public Health, 100*(6), 1019–1028. https://doi.org/10.2105/AJPH.2009.159491
Reich, J. A. (2020). "We are fierce, independent thinkers and intelligent": Social capital and stigma management among mothers who refuse vaccines. *Social Science & Medicine, 257*, 112015. https://doi.org/10.1016/j.socscimed.2018.10.027
Richards, P. (2016). *Ebola: How a people's science helped end an epidemic*. Zed Books.

Riley, K. E., Ulrich, M. R., Hamann, H. A., & Ostroff, J. S. (2017). Decreasing smoking but increasing stigma? Antitobacco campaigns, public health, and cancer care. *AMA Journal of Ethics, 19*(5), 475–485. https://doi.org/10.1001/journalofethics.2017.19.5.msoc1-1705

Rosen, G. (1958). *A history of public health*. The John Hopkins University Press.

Sacks, V. (1996). Women and AIDS: An analysis of media misrepresentations. *Social Science & Medicine, 42*(1), 59–73. https://doi.org/10.1016/0277-9536(95)00079-8

Saguy, A. C., & Alemling, R. (2008). Fat in the fire? Science, the news media, and the « obesity epidemic ». *Sociological Forum, 23*(1), 53–83.

Saguy, A. C., & Gruys, K. (2010). Morality and health: News media constructions of overweight and eating disorders. *Social Problems, 57*(2), 231–250. https://doi.org/10.1525/sp.2010.57.2.231

Scambler, G. (2009). Health-related stigma. *Sociology of Health and Illness, 31*(3), 441–455.

Smith-Morris, C. (2017). Epidemiological placism in public health emergencies: Ebola in two Dallas neighborhoods. *Social Science & Medicine, 179*, 106–114. https://doi.org/10.1016/j.socscimed.2017.02.036

Stevens, R. C., & Hull, S. J. (2013). The colour of AIDS: An analysis of newspaper coverage of HIV/AIDS in the United States from 1992–2007. *Critical Arts, 27*(3), 352–369. https://doi.org/10.1080/02560046.2013.800668

Treichler, P. A. (1988). AIDS, homophobia, and biomedical discourse: An epidemic of signification. In D. Crimp (Ed.), *AIDS: Cultural analysis, cultural activism*. MIT Press.

Wailoo, K. (2006). Stigma, race, and disease in 20th century America. *The Lancet, 367*(9509), 531–533. https://doi.org/10.1016/S0140-6736(06)68186-5

Washer, P. (2010). *Emerging infectious diseases and society*. Palgrave Macmillan.

Wigginton, B., & Lafrance, M. N. (2014). 'I think he is immune to all the smoke I gave him': How women account for the harm of smoking during pregnancy. *Health, Risk & Society, 16*(6), 530–546. https://doi.org/10.1080/13698575.2014.951317

Zylberman, P. (2007). Civilizing the state: Borders, weak states and international health in modern Europe. In A. Bashford (Ed.), *Medicine at the border* (pp. 21–40). Palgrave Macmillan UK. https://doi.org/10.1057/9780230288904_2

6

Social Structures as Determinants of Health Risks

Introduction

Experiences of health risks reveal the strength of social structures. Exposure to danger and resources to avoid or cope with adverse events are not evenly distributed across society. Those with economic, social, and political privileges are less exposed to adverse events and, when they are, their resources allow them to better handle negative outcomes. While global risks do not spare anyone, the COVID-19 pandemic showed how much preexisting inequalities have been exacerbated and not reduced by this public health crisis. Variations in responses to health risks across social groups further illustrate the role of power relations. Some experts define which risks are relevant and which protection measures are legitimate, while they ignore or depreciate concerns raised by people who have less power. This accumulation of advantages and disadvantages, respectively, contributes to reproducing social hierarchies.

In both the social theories of risk and in the medical framing of health risks, social structures are not at the central stage. In this chapter, I aim to show that they play a predominant role across dimensions of health risk experiences since they matter in exposure to risks, in capacities to respond

C. Burton-Jeangros, *Experiences of Health Risks*, Critical Studies in Risk and Uncertainty, https://doi.org/10.1007/978-3-031-65377-3_6

to them and in their interpretations. Both quantitative and qualitative research offer insights into how these social differentiation processes shape experiences of health risks. I address the importance of various social stratification factors, including social class, gender, and ethnic differences, in both interactions and institutional arrangements. The discussion suggests that by not considering the influence of social positions and resources, institutional responses toward risk end up exacerbating social inequalities rather than reducing them.

The overlap between social standing and exposure to risks is very well documented in the health domain since extensive research on health inequalities reveals the tight connections that exist between society and biology. A range of theoretical models aim at revealing the chain of influences through which bodies actually integrate social conditions. They help to understand contrasted exposures to risks across a number of health threats that are socially distributed. Furthermore, research shows how differences in social conditions and exposures influence interpretations and shape responses to danger.

In the first part of the chapter, I present some core elements about social stratification and their consideration in the social theories of risk. I also discuss the theoretical developments associated with the vast literature on health inequalities. The second part draws on empirical findings illustrating the relations between people's positions in society and adverse conditions impacting their health in contexts that often still tend to blame individual behaviors while obliterating structural mechanisms. I also consider how mismatches between experiences and official responses extend into contrasted interpretations of risk and health across categories of the population.

Social Stratification and Health Risks

Basics in Social Stratification

Social stratification, a central preoccupation in sociological theory, focuses on how individuals are positioned in society according to social hierarchies. Since the rise of industrial and capitalist societies, social class based on positions in the labor market has been the dominant factor of stratification. Against the prevailing ideal of social justice, scholars have differently appreciated the importance of inequalities in society, with perspectives oscillating between acute attention to social polarization and others highlighting the overall improvement in living conditions over time and tendencies toward homogenization.

In his foundational work emphasizing the extreme polarization of the emerging industrial society, Karl Marx proposed a conflictual perspective according to the division between manufactures' owners—or bourgeois—and proletarians accomplishing the manual work needed to generate economic value (Grusky, 2019). Despite massive transformations over the twentieth-century working environment, the analysis of class positions by Bourdieu (1979) in France emphasized the strength of social stratification. His propositions, which gained enduring influence, stressed the multidimensionality of social differences through interactions between economic capital, cultural capital, and social capital. He showed that these various forms of resources often overlap; hence, individuals situated at the upper hand of the social spectrum cumulate advantages in material resources, knowledge, and power. In contrast, individuals situated in lower class positions tend to be deprived in all three domains.

In addition to their perspectives, other scholars have stressed homogenizing tendencies as a result of the strengthening of middle-class positions in modern societies. In particular, the economically exceptional postwar period led to theories questioning the relevance of social stratification. To them, the overall improvement of economic conditions and massive shifts of the labor market toward employment in services rather than in industry seemed to reduce social polarization. In an overall optimistic climate, new opportunities in the labor market and the expansion of education were expected to reduce inequalities among future generations. Reduced attention to social stratification was also prompted by rising individualization, which emphasizes the importance of personal agency over the influence of social structures (Pfefferkorn, 2007).

Nevertheless, recurrent economic downturns since the 1970s and globalization forces have reshuffled these perspectives. Academic attention has now turned to increasing social inequalities, both within and across countries. Recent decades saw the increasing accumulation of economic resources and their associated assets, in the hands of the top 1%, a trend documented at the global level (Piketty, 2017). In parallel, it seems that the exceptional trajectories of those born around the 1950s will not be experienced by more recent cohorts (Chauvel, 2002). Hence, aspirations for upper social mobility, which prevailed over the second part of the past century, are now replaced by fears of not being able to maintain the social status gained by one's parents. Therefore, many consider today that social classes remain a central organizing force in society. While they are affected by global socioeconomic transformations, their strength should not be minimized.

Social positions have a widespread influence on society. They affect people's living circumstances through their differentiated access to both material and symbolic resources (Grusky, 2019). These include economic assets gained from work and accumulated wealth, political power or capacity to influence others, cultural capital notably acquired through formal education and informal socialization, and social ties that offer support and access to additional resources. As elaborated below, health is also part of individuals' portfolio of resources. In democratic societies valuing social justice, formal institutions engage in the distribution of resources, for example, through the protection of workers, welfare mechanisms, fiscal redistribution, and universal access to education and health.

While efforts to mitigate inequalities reflect the value attributed to social cohesion, scientists also emphasize the strength of social reproduction. Indeed, social classes should not be considered as isolated entities; rather, they have to be approached in their relations: they exist one against the others. As emphasized by Marx and Bourdieu, they form a system that defines individuals' position and identity compared to other social categories. Those in privileged positions maintain their status by marking their difference from less positioned individuals. They do so through their privileges, allowing them to shape the distribution of resources for others. In addition to their political influence, they informally display their position and privileges through their specific ways of living and values. By marking the frontiers that exist between them and others, they ensure the maintenance and reproduction of their privileges and power. At the same time, those in less favorable positions are constantly encouraged to aspire to a better social status, while everyday circumstances and struggles keep reminding them of the social distance that separates them from privileged positions.

Although debates about social classes have been central in sociology developments, more complex analyses of power in society are currently taking into account other factors shaping social inequalities. The concept of intersectionality was coined in the 1990s to approach the role played by multiple axes of stratification, shaping distinct social locations for individuals, as Crenshaw (1989) claimed that it was necessary to consider the conditions of black women rather than their racial and gender identities separately. Indeed, people simultaneously hold multiple identities that, when combined, generate specific forms of social stratification. Next to gender, race, and social class, other aspects such as age, religion, sexual orientation, dis/ability are considered. Hence, intersectionality aims at shedding light on how individuals are situated within more complex systems of oppression and privileges that affect their life chances. Structural intersectionality considers that institutional arrangements contribute to reproducing divisions in society according to power lines by not paying attention to the specific needs of some individuals (Shields, 2008).

This brief background emphasizes the importance of social stratification across societies and over time. In addition to a general improvement in living conditions, including at the global scale, I consider essential to integrate the persisting and even increasing social polarization between the better and the worse off in the analysis of health risk experiences.

Social Theories of Risks and Inequalities

In the original social theories of risk, authors paid limited attention to the relations between social inequalities and risk. Therefore, the recent *Handbook of Risk and Inequalities* edited by Curran (2022) is a welcome contribution. Indeed, the original social scholarship dedicated to risk in the 1980s–1990s foremost addressed the gap between the positions of experts and reactions in the population, without explicitly addressing social stratification mechanisms. In addition, this literature was produced at a time when the influence of social classes in society was not central to the sociological literature. Nevertheless, some elements of this early social science approach to risk are relevant for this chapter.

Douglas (1990) emphasized how much exposure to danger is shaped by social arrangements when she stated, "The underlying problem in talking about exposure to risk is still justice" (p. 15). Nevertheless, the ideal types elaborated in her cultural analysis do not explicitly associate these positions with social inequalities in society (Olofsson et al., 2014). In his book *Risk Society*, Beck (1992) claimed that the distribution of resources linked to socioeconomic positions in industrial societies was overrun by the distribution of bads at the end of the twentieth century. To him, being exposed to the possibility of catastrophic risks affects everyone's life chance, and no group is able to protect itself from the major threats of the risk society. In his initial writings, he considered that risks, which are increasingly difficult to measure and hence to anticipate, have an equalizing effect across society, as expressed in the quote "poverty is hierarchic, smog is democratic" (p. 36). Beck also talked about a boomerang effect, suggesting that even those behind the production of catastrophic risks would not be able to protect themselves from the harm produced by technologies. He further elaborated his position on increasing individualization, which weakens the sense of class identity through shared life experiences, as was the case in industrial society.

Beck's arguments have been met by criticisms and productive theoretical debates in which Beck took part can be traced (Curran, 2013; Giritli Nygren et al., 2022; Rasborg, 2022). His contradictors emphasized how much vulnerability to risk, notably environmental and financial risks, remains shaped by social class positions; hence, they questioned the equalizing effects of catastrophic risks. Nevertheless, Beck's legacy on that topic should not be undermined (Curran, 2018).

The governmentality perspective inspired by Foucault is interested in how institutions exert power on individuals through technologies of risk surveillance. Ewald (1986) showed how the idea of risk was crucial in the laws put in place in France to compensate for work-related accidents in the industrializing nineteenth-century context and in the establishment of the welfare state. However, over the course of the twentieth century, major demographic and socioeconomic transformations put pressure on welfare regimes (Rasborg, 2022). It appeared that they were unable to respond to expanding new social risks resulting from major social transformations, including the continuous aging of the population, the weakening of traditional gender roles, and the increasing flexibility of labor markets (Ranci, 2010). Giddens (1998, cited in Rasborg, 2022) then considered that these new risks called for a shift from insurance repairing damage to prevention strategies that should avoid the occurrence of harm. Activation policies focused on individual responsibility, observed in unemployment or health (see Chap. 4), indeed reflect such a shift. They expect proactive citizens to self-manage risks when designated as being 'at risk', rather than to claim compensation after damage occurred. These arguments concur with Beck's view that people should not expect protection from institutions; instead, they need to develop personal competencies to deal with pervasive threats (Cebulla, 2007). These perspectives make risk management a personal responsibility, in doing so they often remain silent on how social structures differently affect individuals' vulnerability and capacity to respond to risk (Castel, 2003).

Finally, it is worth mentioning that risk perception research anchored in psychology has paid limited attention to the role of sociological factors in how people assess risks. This quantitative research was conducted through the lens of public understanding of science, focusing on lay-expert gaps. A paper by Boholm (1998) provides a reference for reviewing the evidence about variations in risk perceptions. While he discusses the importance of poverty, which is associated with perceptions of higher risks, he calls for research that would more systematically take into account social stratification factors such as gender, education, and occupation. However, a more recent review of 40 years of risk perception research acknowledges that the focus has remained on the characteristics of the hazards (following the early work of Slovic based on factorial analyses differentiating perceptions of the characteristics of danger), while much less attention has been paid to the characteristics of people evaluating risks (Siegrist & Árvai, 2020).

Authors behind the initial developments in social theories of risk only had a limited engagement with the role of social structures. Accordingly, sparse empirical work has been devoted to studying the interactions between social inequalities and risk (Olofsson et al., 2014). However, interest in the intersection between risk and inequality is developing: "the intensification of the social distribution of risks may not only reproduce class inequalities; it may intensify them" (Curran, 2022, p. 12). Calling for an intersectional risk theory, Olofsson et al. (2014) suggest that it is necessary to jointly examine the extent of risk and of growing inequalities over the past decades. Indeed, they claim that the very modes of risk governance contribute to inequalities. First, the prevailing approaches to risk anchored in technical risk management and psychology make individuals responsible for their own protection irrespective of their differentiated capacity to do so, and thus, they mask the role of structural inequalities. Second, by not considering social structures, formal risk management contributes to reproducing preexisting inequalities and power relationships. It does so by dismissing some reactions toward risk, deemed inadequate, without considering the role that various social markers such as social class, gender, age ethnic origin, or dis/ability can play in the responses elaborated across society. Not paying attention to these social processes evacuates the central role played by moral values in thinking and acting around risks.

Health Inequalities and the Distribution of Risks

After emphasizing that risk and social inequalities have been little considered together, reflecting incompatible research agendas over the end of the twentieth century, I now turn to the theoretical perspective developed around health, risks, and inequalities.

While they were at the core of public health initiatives during the nineteenth century, social inequalities in health were then long eclipsed as a result of the success of modern medicine. Over the first part of the twentieth century, the idea prevailed that access to medical treatment would offer equal chances for everyone to be in good health. This optimistic vision overlapped with the prosperous postwar period, during which socioeconomic inequalities tended to decline and were thus little addressed.

Both social and health inequalities came back on scientific and political agendas over the last third of the past century. A number of sharp critiques toward medicine emerged in the 1970s, newly characterized by increasing costs, excessive medicalization, and the limitations of medical treatments in a shifting landscape of diseases (Illich, 1975). The need to focus attention on good health rather than disease was at the heart of the new public health movement (Petersen & Lupton, 1996), initiated with the landmark report of Marc Lalonde, Health Minister, in 1974 'A new perspective on the health of Canadians'. This innovative framework geared attention toward prevention by highlighting that a range of health determinants matter: beyond biology through individuals' genetic make-up and access to health care, the role of the social and physical environment as well as individual behaviors through health-related lifestyles was emphasized. It was followed by the development of health promotion under the influence of the World Health Organization in the 1980s.

In parallel, mounting evidence has confirmed that social factors definitely affect individuals' health status. Following the pioneering work conducted in the United Kingdom with the Black report in 1980, a social gradient in health started to be systematically observed across contexts. This gradient refers to the fact that for each step gained in the social hierarchy, be it measured by social class, income, or education, individual health status improves (Marmot, 2004). The international acknowledgment of these inequalities led to the establishment of the World Health Organization Commission on Social Determinants of Health in 2005. Its report 'Closing the gap in a generation' (Marmot et al., 2008) stressed the pervasiveness of the social gradient in health at the global scale while developing policy propositions to address these inequalities.

According to epidemiological reasoning focused on the distribution of population health, such inequalities reflect differentiated exposures to risks. A central issue then consists in the definition of which risks need to be identified and addressed. Accordingly, a number of competing explanatory models have been formulated since the 1980s, striving to clarify how social inequalities "get under people's skin" (Ferraro & Shippee, 2009). As presented below, the formulation of these different models reflects continuing debates across disciplines regarding the roles of biological and social determinants, respectively.

In medicine, genome sequencing techniques have recently attracted massive funding to support precision or personalized medicine, which promises to tailor treatments based on individual genetic make-up.

However, the contributions of these developments to population health are questioned since nongenetic factors would outweigh the role of genes in health (Vermeulen et al., 2020). In addition, social scientists have been particularly critical of genetic determinism (Arribas-Ayllon, 2016), which has been used in the past to explain variations in health. Following historical infamous episodes, references to biological or genetic criteria to explain poverty or social unworthiness and to justify the formulation of eugenic policies have been severely criticized. At the same time, excluding the biological underpinning of differences in health is currently considered inadequate (Harris & Schorpp, 2018); this exclusion is notably contradicted by developments in epigenetics showing the complex interplay occurring between biological and social conditions. Therefore, biosocial approaches are currently advocated for analyzing the interactions that exist between genes, behaviors, and the environment. Recent developments around the concept of embodiment invite us to examine how the individual body incorporates social and ecological circumstances in a dynamic manner, while adopting a perspective that challenges genetic essentialism (Kelly-Irving & Delpierre, 2021).

The broad concept of the exposome was coined to counterbalance the growing importance attributed by some researchers to the genome. It shifts the attention to the environmental drivers of health and disease, that is, to nongenetic factors, encompassing a large range of risks susceptible to affecting health (Vermeulen et al., 2020). Indeed, the long absence of an ecosystemic perspective on health is considered regrettable (Cicolella, 2017), especially when one considers that the burden of noncommunicable diseases developed over decades characterized by an increasing chemical pollution.

Despite the role played by a number of activists, such as Rachel Carson in her book Silent Spring published in 1962, the environment indeed long remained a black box for epidemiology. In addition to local evidence gathered by concerned people activists and sometimes further explored by social scientists, systematic research on environmental influences on population health remains limited. Next to the data and methodological challenges associated with analyzing the complex relationships between multiple and cumulative exposures and individual health (Vermeulen et al., 2020), it is observed that exposome research has so far paid limited attention to the role of social factors in environmental exposure (Neufcourt et al., 2022).

Since the association between socioeconomic conditions and the distribution of disease is an enduring phenomenon, observed across time and place despite important transformations in diseases and in factors that expose or protect individuals, sociologists theorized about the mechanisms through which social health inequalities are reproduced. The fundamental cause theory (Clouston & Link, 2021; Link & Phelan, 1995) proposes moving away from the proximate factors, typically behaviors integrated into epidemiological models, to look at the distant social factors that shape health. Considering that inequalities are particularly large in preventable conditions, this perspective emphasizes the importance of access to a large range of resources since privileged people are systematically more able to avoid being sick. Protective resources, including money, knowledge, power, prestige, and social connections, are all associated with better health. Hence, their uneven distribution in society helps explain the persistence of health inequalities across contexts and over time.

Intersectionality has been introduced in health inequality research to consider how people's lives and health are simultaneously shaped by their multiple social identities. Indeed, systematic health disparities are observed according to a number of social stratification factors. Hence, intersectionality is mobilized to better understand health inequalities in the context of the circumstances experienced by people as a result of the overlap between their socioeconomic position, gender, and race (Gkiouleka et al., 2018). This approach moves beyond analyses of how single attributes impact individuals' health to consider the processes that shape and reproduce health inequalities through the complex embodiment of multiple identities.

Considering that social positions are relational implies that the privileges of some exist because of the disadvantages of others, and reciprocally. How efforts to maintain one's place in society contribute to the stigmatization of others was discussed in Chap. 5. The combination of stigma, experiences of stress, and social disadvantage contributes to poorer health. It has been proposed that lower income groups are more likely to experience a sense of 'shame, inferiority and subordination' as a result of prevailing narratives about social worth (Marmot & Wilkinson,

1999). In other words, interactions across social groups contribute to the greater vulnerability of those situated in lower positions relative to others. The effects of such social dynamic were observed in the early days of the HIV epidemic, when Jonathan Mann (1997), then director of the WHO Global Programme on AIDS, stated that "as the HIV epidemic matures and evolves within each community and country, it focuses inexorably on those groups who, before HIV/AIDS arrived, were already discriminated against, marginalized, and stigmatized within each society" (p. 10).

Approaching privileges and disadvantages as the result of a power system that distributes resources differently also encourages researchers to pay attention to institutional arrangements. Indeed, in its multiple layers, the social determinants of health framework points to the role played by societal structures in exposure or protection from health risks. Institutions define which categories of people need attention when other groups are marginalized (Gkiouleka et al., 2018). In their discussion of the role played by institutions, Frohlich & Potvin (2008) emphasize the shortcomings of standard population approaches in health prevention. Indeed, universal perspectives which do not address the underlying mechanisms shaping exposure to risks contribute to exacerbating differences across social groups since more privileged people benefit more from prevention strategies. The authors then advocate a vulnerable population approach, different from population or at-risk group campaigns that target single risk factors. A vulnerable population is defined by being at "higher risk of risks" due to its social characteristics. This invites to consider how vulnerable groups' health is shaped through the combination of life course influences and concentrations of risks: "Vulnerable populations, we argue, are those who concentrate numerous risk factors throughout their life course because of shared fundamental causes associated with their position in the social structure" (p. 219).

The dynamic character of health underlies the development of life course epidemiology since the 1990s (Burton-Jeangros, 2020; Burton-Jeangros et al., 2015). It aims at understanding the unfolding of individual trajectories within their specific temporal and spatial locations. Considering the importance of age, cohorts, and historic periods helps to understand the different types of risks individuals encounter with regard to their health. These exposures reflect both changing morbidity and mortality patterns but also transformations in technology, demography, and economics, which all matter for individual and population health. This means that health risks have to be considered within specific contexts, which redefine not only actual risks but also their interpretations and the measures put in place to prevent them. Considering that health is a dynamic process, people's current health is determined by successive layers of past circumstances. In addition, each cohort has been exposed to contrasted risks (e.g., the balance between noncommunicable and infectious diseases), but also to changing preventive norms. Besides emphasizing the accumulation of advantages or disadvantages over the individual life course, this perspective highlights the importance of approaching the determinants that shape people's health in both individual time and collective time.

With this first section of the chapter, I aimed at presenting the theoretical developments around social stratification, risk, and health that help to understand the differences across social groups as a result of their contrasted resources. In the next section, I present a range of findings showing how they matter in experiences of health risks.

Empirical Evidence on Health Risks and Social Inequalities

Empirical findings addressing the connection between social stratification and health inequalities describe how exposure and then responses to risks are structurally organized. First, the social science literature dedicated to health risks offers insights into socially differentiated exposures to risks in relation to the environments where people live and work. I wish to contrast the dominant risk framework which tends to focus on risk characteristics, notably in the domain of health, with a social science perspective inviting to consider people's characteristics. Second, I discuss how responses to risks are shaped by socially situated systems of values, challenging assumptions that health risk prevention models are neutral or based on values uniformly endorsed across social categories.

Socially Differentiated Exposures and Communities at Risk

The pervasiveness of health inequalities suggests that, across social contexts, the burden of risks is not equally shared across society. Health inequalities indicate that social classes have not lost their relevance in the risk society. In the case of major public health events, such as the COVID-19 pandemic, socially vulnerable people were more likely to suffer. Different streams of research document how some groups of the population are more systematically and extensively exposed to conditions harming their health and how these are more often characterized by their limited power in society.

Social Determinants of Health Inequalities

The social epidemiology perspective calls for analyses of the distribution of health in the population, and empirical findings systematically show the poorer health status of those in less advantaged social positions. This suggests that exposures to risks impacting health are socially differentiated. These observations are robust, independent of the health or social position indicators used. However, this research has long ignored how people's multiple social characteristics jointly affect their chances of living long and in good health.

Indeed, initial evidence on health inequalities reflects the long-standing focus of sociological and medical research on men while paying limited attention to women's social and health-specific circumstances. However, in both respects, women are not equivalent to men. First, the former remain on average in subordinate social positions compared to men, as notably assessed by their lower incomes. Second, they live longer than men but report poorer health throughout their life course. As an illustration, our analyses conducted with Swiss data showed the importance of considering both work and family roles, especially since family circumstances affect men and women differently, with a notable impact of being a single parent on women's mental health (Burton-Jeangros, 2009; Burton-Jeangros & Rinaldi, 2008). Recent research has gone further by considering how gender generates differences between men's and women's health at multiple social layers through the concept of structural sexism (Homan, 2019). Homan's findings show that sexism does not matter at the individual level when it is assessed with personal views about women's roles. However, meso-level sexism (measured by inequality in marital relations) and macrolevel sexism (measured by systematic gender inequality at the state level) affect women's and men's health status in different ways. These results confirm the importance of examining how distant determinants, beyond behaviors, affect the multiple risks impacting people's health.

Findings in life course epidemiology add a dynamic perspective since they consider how variations in living circumstances, including family and work roles, are related to variations in health (Cullati, 2014; Cullati et al., 2014). A systematic review of this domain revealing that women's trajectories tend to be more complex than men's trajectories shows that early transition to parenthood, single parenthood, and weak ties to employment are related to women's poorer health, while those with a longer education, stronger ties to the labor market, and later parenthood overall report better health outcomes (Machů et al., 2022).

Indeed, the accumulation of large databases of longitudinal data collected across countries provides additional possibilities for understanding how health opportunities are related to institutional contexts. Analyses have shown, for example, that greater gender stratification is related to larger inequalities in cancer screening across women's education levels (Willems et al., 2020), that better access to health care and social protection mitigates cancer screening inequalities (De Prez et al., 2022; Jolidon et al., 2021), and that greater social protection expenditures could attenuate inequalities in various health outcomes (Sieber et al., 2021). These findings provide empirical evidence on the relevance of an institutional perspective that considers "the welfare state as an institutional arrangement—a set of 'rules of the game'—that distributes health" (Beckfield et al., 2015, p. 227).

In addition, the accumulation of longitudinal data allows for analyses of trajectories of unequal aging, combining concepts from both the life course and intersectionality perspectives (Holman & Walker, 2021). Beyond the role of social class and gender in the distribution of health risks, inequalities with respect to race and ethnicity are also systematically observed. The concept of structural racism developed in the United States to take into account “the totality of ways in which societies foster racial discrimination, through mutually reinforcing inequitable systems (in housing, education, employment, earnings, benefits, credit, media, health care, criminal justice, and so on) that in turn reinforce discriminatory beliefs, values, and distribution of resources, which together affect the risk of adverse health outcomes” (Bailey et al., 2017, p. 1454). This suggests that current inequalities are associated with the long reach of past practices of colonialism, slavery, and racism as experienced over individuals' life course and across generations. While experiences of sexism, ageism, and racism change over historical time (Holman & Walker, 2021), health inequality research indicates that despite these variations, those in unprivileged positions keep being exposed to more risks affecting their health status across periods.

This brief overview of an expanding domain of research confirms that social inequalities are related to health disparities. I showed that the social determinants of health perspective suggests that detrimental risk exposures are socially structured through unequal access to material and symbolic resources that can protect against these adverse exposures. The interdependence between biological and social factors questions the biomedical perspective tackling health risks through the lens of biology or behaviors. The robustness and complexity of health inequalities reveal the importance of biosocial mechanisms, encompassing environmental factors that challenge the responsibility of individuals with regard to their health status. In the next two sections, I present how medical anthropology documented these mechanisms and how its contributions help to understand the difficulty for people who are exposed to social and environmental risks to be acknowledged in their experiences.

Syndemics and Biosocial Mechanisms

Another way to consider differential exposure to risk factors for disease emerged with the concept of syndemics, coined in the 1990s (Singer & Clair, 2003), in the context of the HIV/AIDS epidemic. Adopting a critical medical anthropology perspective, the goal was to address the social and medical conditions typically co-occurring in HIV-infected people (Mendenhall et al., 2022). Three rules are associated with the concept of syndemics: first, two or more diseases co-occur; second, these clusters are related to social, psychological, and biological factors that interact; and third, these interactions are exacerbated by social conditions. This perspective not only connects biological and social factors, but also integrates the importance of social inequalities. This concept is clearly innovative in challenging the classical biomedical perspective, which focuses on diseases as discrete and objective entities that are separate from other pathologies, as well as from the groups or contexts in which they occur (Singer & Clair, 2003). Stressing that diseases do not occur in a social vacuum, biosocial approaches encompass interrelationships and influences from the environment in which people live, since it is commonly observed that comorbidities and adverse social conditions cluster.

Over the years, the concept has expanded and gained visibility in public health and medicine. When the COVID-19 pandemic emerged, it was used by social scientists to question the assumption, commonly shared by politicians and in the media, that the virus would impact everyone equally (Bambra et al., 2020). Such an assumption has been challenged over the development of the pandemic since evidence confirmed that COVID-19 morbidity and mortality were related to social factors, with disadvantaged social groups being more seriously impacted, such as ethnic minorities in the United States (Bambra et al., 2020). The socioeconomic consequences of the virus were more broadly documented with interviews conducted across six European countries revealing 'a second pandemic' following social hierarchies, hence stressing the strength of structural inequality (Fiske et al., 2022).

Indeed, the pandemic confirmed the importance of considering biosocial mechanisms (Singer & Rylko-Bauer, 2021). The virus had more severe consequences among people who suffer from preexisting chronic conditions, such as diabetes, hypertension, and asthma. It is well established from health inequality research that these conditions are more prevalent among already socially disadvantaged people. It turned out that "The theory of syndemics is relevant for understanding the pandemic because COVID-19 demonstrates affliction due to both disease concentration and disease interaction driven by harmful social conditions" (Mendenhall et al., 2022, p. 114655). Being exposed to occupational risks, more frequent among essential workers delivering first-line services (e.g., healthcare, commerce), living in disadvantaged neighborhoods, being a member of minority groups, and having differential access to healthcare all played a role in COVID-19 morbidity and mortality (Singer & Rylko-Bauer, 2021). In its far-reaching approach, the concept of syndemics also invites us to pay attention to psychosocial pathways, including stress related to subordinate social positions and experiences of stigma, as part of the synergies that impact upon health (Singer et al., 2017). Finally, some researchers suggested that public health measures themselves contributed to the socially differentiated impact of the pandemic, with job and income loss or overcrowding during lockdowns being more detrimental for less privileged people.

It is, however, important to emphasize that the capacity to document these biosocial mechanisms empirically has been impaired by the kind of data that were routinely collected. Indeed, in Switzerland, as elsewhere, it turned out that only limited data were collected on the social stratification factors of COVID-19 infections and their consequences. Researchers had to develop innovative strategies to assess socially differentiated effects through, for example, a neighborhood deprivation index based on people's postal addresses (Mongin et al., 2022; Riou et al., 2021). This means that most vulnerable groups typically remained off the institutional radar. It was only because we were at that time already conducting a longitudinal study on irregular migrants living in Geneva that we had the opportunity to collect data on their specific conditions during the first weeks of the lockdown in spring 2020. These analyses showed the considerable impact of the pandemic and public health measures on this previously vulnerable population, impacting their capacity to work in the domestic sector, threatening their housing in the absence of income, and generating food insecurity (Burton-Jeangros et al., 2020).

Research efforts combining theoretical developments with both qualitative and quantitative data analyses are thus essential to better understand the complexity of the mechanisms leading to differentiated risk exposures. These mechanisms are shaped not only by conditions of the social environment but also by interactions across social groups.

Dangerous Environments

I wish to integrate a third domain of research that illustrates the unequal exposure to risk, moving the focus to dangerous environmental circumstances, in the occupational and ecological domains. Developments in these domains are recent, reflecting the difficulty of assessing the impact of environmental exposure on health over time due to multiple exposures and delayed effects. While the importance of environmental exposures is now more systematically integrated into health policy strategies, evidence remains limited.

The role of environmental risks was acknowledged as a result of the pressure of exposed communities in the United States in the 1980s. Environmental justice has since been adopted by the Environmental Protection Agency (EPA) with the following definition: "fair treatment and meaningful involvement of all people regardless of race, skin color, national origin and income with respect to the development, implementation and enforcement of laws, regulations and environmental policies (EPA, 2014)" (Di Fonzo et al., 2022, p. 114834). With an emphasis on environmental distributive justice, these authors performed a systematic review of the literature to assess what is currently known about the distribution of health hazards from polluting facilities with a focus on social inequalities. Their review concluded that available findings confirm that exposure to pollution sources is unequally distributed across society, with ethnic minorities and economically vulnerable communities being more at risk. However, the existing evidence offers only limited evaluations of the impact of this pollution on individuals' health.

As observed by Wynne (1996) decades ago already, the absence of quantified evidence is a major issue. Findings from anthropological case studies describing the chemical exposures of socially disadvantaged communities have been instrumental in raising awareness about environmental risks. For example, social scientists have documented the impact of manufactured risks, such as the 'cancer alley' or 'chemical corridor' situated in the southern United States (Singer, 2011) or the shanty town surrounded by the largest petrochemical compound in Argentina (Auyero & Swistun, 2008). They emphasize how dominant or official narratives—from both the government and the industry—regularly dismissed the existence of environmental risks for these populations, even in the case of elevated cases of death or disease. Another case study on exposure to occupational risks (Adams et al., 2023) investigated the possible connection between elevated cases of lupus and regular exposure to agricultural chemicals among black women working as farmworkers in Florida. In that case, again, the relation has been contested by institutions, including medical doctors and politicians, devaluing the workers' claims based on their concrete experiences. A study on workers' exposure to pesticides in France similarly reports on how institutions emphasize faulty individual behaviors as the source of intoxication, with workers' failure to correctly use the protective equipment, without questioning the adequacy of this equipment (Jouzel & Dedieu, 2013). Such moral judgments make it particularly difficult for workers to report their exposure to risks.

Krieger et al. (2008) proposed referring to such risk exposures with the inverse hazard law: "The accumulation of health hazards tends to vary inversely with the power and resources of the populations affected" (p. 1971). While the authors acknowledged the methodological issues related to testing this inverse hazard law, notably since small sample sizes limit the capacity to establish environmental or occupational risks, they stress that the low number of cases should not be a sufficient reason to dismiss exposures. This tension between lay experiences on the one hand and scientific and policy framings on the other hand has been approached with the concept of 'popular epidemiology' (Brown, 1987). It conflicts with experts' reliance on statistical significance, which is required to establish evidence but necessitates an elevated number of occurrences.

Overall, a number of qualitative studies have reported that it remains common for officials, experts, or stakeholders in private industries to refer to behavioral and individualistic approaches to risks. This allows them to dismiss the claims that their industry or the associated working conditions are harmful. Indeed, not only are environmental determinants dismissed, but claims for alternative models "are often met with derision, anger, disbelief, and even ridicule" (Adams et al., 2023, p. 3). The dismissal of the adverse experiences of disadvantaged people contributes to the reproduction of social hierarchies, exacerbating the feelings of powerlessness of those who are situated at the lower end of social prestige. Singer (2011) reported on such feelings explicitly expressed by local residents of the Cancer alley; when they declared in interviews that as "small people", they could not compete with "Big Men" sitting in offices and representing the government.

With the elements presented in this section, I show the tight connections that exist between being exposed to a range of risks (viruses, chemical substances, and catastrophes) and groups of people who are situated at the lower end of social hierarchies. Their experiences are constantly depreciated and interpreted within the prevailing risk management framework, which, in addition, questions the differential responses people adopt when confronted with danger.

Socially Differentiated Responses to Risk

Research on social representations of illness and health, notably initiated by Herzlich (1992) in France in the 1960s, emphasizes the multiple understandings that coexist in society about these entities. In this section, I address some elements about the social structuring of representations of risk, which contribute to explaining the persisting differences across groups of the population faced with adversity.

Interpretations of Risk

Fundamental cause theory proposes that resources are important for protecting people's health (Link & Phelan, 1995). In addition, they affect their interpretations of the dangers they are exposed to. Across issues, evidence suggests that those with less power in society tend to perceive risks as higher than those who have more privileges. Studies on risk understandings in recent public health crises, related, for example, to interpretations of nuclear risk after the Fukushima accident or infectious risks in the context of the COVID-19 pandemic, have provided relevant insights. Indeed, crises represent particularly heuristic contexts in which it is possible to assess how people perceive risks under 'unsettled circumstances' (Swidler, 1986).

Some research highlighted a 'white male effect', reflecting the combined role of gender and race in understandings of risk: white men would rate risks as lower than any other social group (Finucane et al., 2000). There is however today limited consensus in the literature about the role of different social stratification factors on risk perceptions (Giritli Nygren et al., 2022). Some findings suggest that "power, control, and vulnerability are key mechanisms that shape perceived risk" (Umamaheswar & Tan, 2020, p. 2). In this qualitative study, men's and women's COVID-19 risk perceptions were equivalent, but women expressed more concern and fear. The authors attributed this difference to the gendered division of labor and, notably, the sense of responsibility people have toward others, which tends to be significantly different between men and women. Similar findings have been reported in situations of environmental exposure to risks, such as studies dedicated to understanding nuclear exposure in the aftermath of the Fukushima accident in 2011. Women, especially mothers, perceived risks as higher than men and were particularly preoccupied about the effects of the catastrophe on physical health, their own and their children's, with preoccupations centered on food (Morioka, 2014). Their concerns were dismissed by their husbands and by officials, who were more trusted by men. These contrasted reactions to the nuclear catastrophe generated tensions within households, with men regretting their wives' emotional reactions, considering them "irrational, neurotic, or obsessive".

Other studies have emphasized how the privileges associated with race positions are also important for understanding risk. In the United States, Vargas et al. (2023) reported quantitative findings indicating that race was a predominant factor in evaluations of COVID-19 risk, with racialized minorities feeling more vulnerable to the virus. They suggest that "white privilege manifests as a protective cultural lens that filters out the fears, anxieties, and vulnerabilities that individuals might encounter in unsettled moments" (p. 2). Having more resources and privileges is often associated with greater trust in institutions but also with fewer past adverse experiences.

These elements reflect the long absence of social characteristics in risk perception research (Siegrist & Árvai, 2020). However, they confirm that risk consciousness develops in situated settings in which people are aware (and repeatedly made aware by others, as I show in Chap. 5) of their position amidst power dynamics (Giritli Nygren & Olofsson, 2014). Overall, being in a position characterized by fewer resources is likely to increase feelings of vulnerability.

Understandings of Health

The social distribution of health practices is well documented. Less systematic attention has been paid to the role played by people's contrasted understandings of health and risk in their differential adoption of preventive practices. The public health norms rest on a number of assumptions, including the fact that people value their health and their capacity to control risks but also that they endorse a long-term perspective that convinces them to act today for their health in the future. However, findings suggest that these assumptions do not echo the experiences and understandings of risks across society.

The values of control and projection to the future are indeed typical of the middle classes: "the goal of health became an essential component of what it meant to be modern, progressive, rational, and distinctive" (Crawford, 1994, p. 1349). The logic described by Weber (1964 [1904]) in his discussion of ascetism and the importance attributed to savings for future gains can be valued by those who have reached a certain security in life. This allows them to move beyond preoccupations related to primary needs and immediate concerns and to direct their efforts toward expected future gains. In parallel to economic savings, preventive efforts are driven by an orientation to the future: today's investments in health are expected to provide later benefits.

Bourdieu's concept of habitus, connecting lifestyles and class positions, suggests that tastes and dispositions are socially shaped through socialization. Social groups characterized by lower levels of resources focus on 'choices of necessity' and immediate concerns, which means that they have a lower capacity and willingness to anticipate the future than more privileged social categories. These elements can be related to attitudes toward health risks through 'embodied dispositions' interested in how class tastes materialize in the body (Boltanksi, 1971). This important text proposed a distinction between an instrumental relation to the body and to health, focused on present necessities to conduct one's life, as opposed to an expressive relation to the body and to health, approaching them as personal projects to be constantly worked on. These considerations suggest that the willingness to prevent health risks depends on people's perception of their capacity to actually control their present health and their social conditions (Savage et al., 2013).

In a qualitative study with underprivileged men undergoing cardiac rehabilitation in Canada, concepts of short-termism and fatalism emerged inductively from the interviews: participants emphasized their lack of control over everyday stress in the context of lives characterized by economic precarity (Savage et al., 2013). The authors proposed to situate their difficulties or reluctance to plan for the future, and hence to modify their health practices, within their general sense of powerlessness and vulnerability. Those men who had a sense of their shorter-than-average life expectancy (according to their past health and reflecting health inequalities) preferred to focus on the present and prioritized their quality of life over unlikely long-term gains. Another qualitative study with young obese women living in underprivileged conditions similarly emphasized their primary focus on immediate needs and responsibilities, especially among mothers toward their children (Dumas et al., 2014). Their limited resources, in terms of money and time, combined with the stress of their everyday life prevented them from endorsing obesity prevention messages. A comparison of overweight women from middle and lower social classes further confirmed the importance of orientation to the future and perceptions of control over one's life circumstances: "Investments in long-term health are the outcome of socially constructed tastes and preferences, distinctive time horizons, and values given to its perceived advantages" (Audet et al., 2017, p. 1549).

These findings reveal that less privileged social lives tend to be organized around more short-term issues. The capacity to work and earn a living being central to health is approached from an instrumental and functional perspective: the body is foremost perceived in terms of its capacity to work. This was confirmed in our study on undocumented migrants in Geneva, accumulating unfavorable circumstances through the absence of a legal status as a result of migration, being female and employed in domestic work. The findings show the impact of undocumented work on their deteriorated mental health, while most still reported good self-reported health despite their difficult and dangerous living and occupational conditions (Refle et al., 2023). This gap can be attributed to their situated understanding of health, which more broadly offered them little room for health practices oriented toward long-term objectives and made risk prevention less relevant.

Projections toward the future and the relevance of investing in health gains in the distant future are affected by previous social experiences, which vary across social categories. Previous experiences of adversity and vulnerability are hence likely to hamper the willingness to tackle risks. They also explain why references to fatalism, destiny, luck, or fate, contesting the official narrative of illness as being controllable through individual efforts, remain important in some social categories (Davison et al., 1992). These aspects are important in two respects: on the one hand, they contribute to explaining why social position matters in the adoption of preventive recommendations; on the other hand, they emphasize the situated character of these norms, formulated by professionals in privileged social positions who assume that their own values apply universally. These results invite to pay attention to the co-presence of multiple understandings of risk and vulnerability in society. In addition to official definitions, people's understandings are shaped by their everyday social experiences and interactions (Burton-Jeangros & Fargnoli, 2023).

Conclusion

This chapter aimed to show how, by not paying sufficient attention to the role of social structures, research and policy focusing on the characteristics of health risks may often reinforce inequalities.

Indeed, social structures affect experiences of health risks. The robust social gradient in health evidences the tight connections existing between social and health inequalities. It indicates that the way society is structurally organized according to social and economic hierarchies results in systematic variations in exposure to risks. References to the social determinants of health are nowadays commonplace still, across disciplines and domains, this approach remains constantly challenged by research and lay interpretations focused on individual factors, from genetic make-up to health behaviors.

Hence, despite the increasing evidence about such differentiated exposures, the socially differentiated harm of occupational or environmental risks is still denied, as these observations remain difficult to integrate into the formal risk management model. In the absence of findings based on sufficiently large numbers and/or of socially stratified analyses, local experiences of harm are challenged or attributed to individuals' wrongdoing. These conflicting views reflect the gap between a perspective focused on how people experience risks, especially as is documented in qualitative studies, and an approach centered on the technical or material characteristics of the risk that pays little attention to how it interacts with people's local circumstances.

At the same time, studies suggest that people who are more exposed to risks are actually aware of their higher-than-average exposure. They reported feeling more vulnerable than more privileged people as a result of their lower capacity to control their actual living circumstances. This extends into health and social trajectories marked by greater adversity, which impacts their appraisals of risks and, in particular, their perception of their own capacity to mitigate them through their own actions. Therefore, despite their more acute sense of vulnerability, they do not endorse healthy behavior recommendations that do not make sense to them in the face of the multiple external threats they are exposed to without having control of them.

This relates to the observation that health prevention programs might increase health inequalities through differentiated adherence to prevention norms. These norms are aligned with middle- and upper-classes values toward investing in the future through personal efforts. In parallel, the incompatibility between these norms and the difficulties encountered by people living in disadvantaged circumstances can reinforce defiance toward recommendations focused on individual risk, while broader problems of unprivileged living conditions are not addressed. In Chap. 5, I tackled these processes in the discussion about conspiracy views.

The role of pervasive social stratification mechanisms extends into conditions that affect physical and mental health, as observed in the systematically lower health statuses of groups in dominated positions. This confirms the necessity of addressing the conditions of vulnerable populations who are "at higher risk of risks" (Frohlich & Potvin, 2008) and focusing on distant rather than proximate determinants of health (Clouston & Link, 2021). This calls for an agenda addressing risks in all policies, not only in health policies, as advocated in many contexts. The implementation of this agenda, however, remains difficult. The tight overlap that people experience in the relations between their socioeconomic and health concerns is not aligned with the way welfare institutions have been organized since the mid-twentieth century. The deliberate separation between social and health policies at that time deeply shaped the institutional landscape (Duvoux & Vezinat, 2023). Today, it continues to impact strategies developed to address social and health risks.

Another important insight gained with this chapter is that in many instances, the situated character of prevention is not sufficiently discussed. Messages and recommendations reflect the values of health professionals or experts who occupy privileged positions in social hierarchies. Their thinking and actions about health risks are affected by their resources and living conditions, which are quite different from those of other, less advantaged segments of society. When this is not acknowledged, the distance between social groups is accentuated, especially when top-down judgments reinforce the illegitimacy of noncompliant responses. This disqualifies people situated in lower social positions in their understandings and contributes to stress and stigmatization as drivers of poor health. These processes are made visible in instances when experiences of inequalities expand into feelings of injustice and social mobilization. However, next to those who manage to engage in social mobilization and have their position heard, many remain silent and invisible.

The role of social structures discussed in this chapter has two important implications for the social theories of risk. First, it shows that it is most relevant to approach the relations between risk and social inequalities, as adverse experiences exacerbate previous hierarchies in society. Second, ignoring these mechanisms keep power relations invisible. Nevertheless, those who are situated in lower social positions are constantly reminded of their marginal and illegitimate status in society which makes them feel both powerless and more vulnerable.

References

Adams, A. E., Saville, A., & Shriver, T. E. (2023). Race, toxic exposures, and environmental health: The contestation of lupus among farmworkers. *Journal of Health and Social Behavior, 64*(1), 136–151. https://doi.org/10.1177/00221465221132787

Arribas-Ayllon, M. (2016). After geneticization. *Social Science & Medicine, 159*, 132–139. https://doi.org/10.1016/j.socscimed.2016.05.011

Audet, M., Dumas, A., Binette, R., & Dionne, I. J. (2017). Lifestyle inequalities: Explaining socioeconomic differences in preventive practices of clinically overweight women after menopause. *Qualitative Health Research, 27*(10), 1541–1552. https://doi.org/10.1177/1049732317715246

Auyero, J., & Swistun, D. (2008). The social production of toxic uncertainty. *American Sociological Review, 73*(3), 357–379.

Bailey, Z. D., Krieger, N., Agénor, M., Graves, J., Linos, N., & Bassett, M. T. (2017). Structural racism and health inequities in the USA: Evidence and interventions. *The Lancet, 389*(10077), 1453–1463. https://doi.org/10.1016/S0140-6736(17)30569-X

Bambra, C., Riordan, R., Ford, J., & Matthews, F. (2020). The COVID-19 pandemic and health inequalities. *Journal of Epidemiology and Community Health, 74*(11), 964. https://doi.org/10.1136/jech-2020-214401

Beck, U. (1992). *Risk society. Towards a new modernity*. Sage. [1986: first edition in German *Risikogesellschaft*].

Beckfield, J., Bambra, C., Eikemo, T. A., Huijts, T., McNamara, C., & Wendt, C. (2015). An institutional theory of welfare state effects on the distribution of population health. *Social Theory & Health, 13*(3), 227–244. https://doi.org/10.1057/sth.2015.19

Boholm, A. (1998). Comparative studies of risk perception: A review of twenty years of research. *Journal of Risk Research, 1*(2), 135–163.

Boltanksi, L. (1971). Les usages sociaux du corps. *Annales Economies, Sociétés, Civilisations, 26e*(1), 205–233.

Bourdieu, P. (1979). *La distinction: Critique sociale du jugement.* Éditions de Minuit.
Brown, M. S. (1987). Communicating information about workplace hazards: Effects on worker attitudes toward risks. In B. B. Johnson & V. T. Covello (Eds.), *The social construction of risk: Essays on risk selection and perception.* D. Reidel Publishing.
Burton-Jeangros, C. (2009). Les inégalités face à la santé: L'impact des trajectoires familiales et professionnelles sur les hommes et les femmes. In M. Oris, E. Widmer, A. de Ribeaupierre, D. Joye, D. Spini, G. Labouvie-Vief, & J.-M. Falter (Eds.), *Transitions dans les parcours de vie et construction des inégalités* (pp. 273–295). Presses polytechniques et universitaires romandes.
Burton-Jeangros, C. (2020). Life course approaches in global health. In R. Haring, I. Kickbusch, D. Ganten, & M. Moeti (Eds.), *Handbook of global health* (pp. 1–28). Springer International Publishing. https://doi.org/10.1007/978-3-030-05325-3_42-1
Burton-Jeangros, C., Cullati, S., Sacker, A., & Blane, D. (Eds.). (2015). *A life course perspective on health trajectories and transitions* (Vol. 4). Springer International Publishing. https://doi.org/10.1007/978-3-319-20484-0
Burton-Jeangros, C., Duvoisin, A., Lachat, S., Consoli, L., Fakhoury, J., & Jackson, Y. (2020). The impact of the Covid-19 Pandemic and the lockdown on the health and living conditions of undocumented migrants and migrants undergoing legal status regularization. *Frontiers in Public Health, 8*, 940. https://doi.org/10.3389/fpubh.2020.596887
Burton-Jeangros, C., & Fargnoli, V. (2023). Vulnerability around health issues: Trajectories, experiences and meanings. In D. Spini & E. Widmer (Eds.), *Withstanding vulnerability throughout adult life* (pp. 189–204). Springer Nature Singapore. https://doi.org/10.1007/978-981-19-4567-0_12
Burton-Jeangros, C., & Rinaldi, J.-M. (2008). Santé des mères élevant seules leurs enfants. In M. Katharina (Ed.), *La santé en Suisse. Rapport national sur la santé 2008* (pp. 63–74). Médecine & Hygiène.
Castel, R. (2003). *L'insécurité sociale: Qu'est-ce qu'être protégé?* Seuil.
Cebulla, A. (2007). Class or individual? A test of the nature of risk perceptions and the individualisation thesis of risk society theory. *Journal of Risk Research, 10*(2), 129–148. https://doi.org/10.1080/13669870601066948
Chauvel, L. (2002). *Le destin des générations: Structure sociale et cohortes en France au XXe siècle* (2nd ed.). Presses Universitaires de France.
Cicolella, A. (2017). Le trente-troisième anniversaire de la santé environnementale. *Les Tribunes de la santé, 54*(1), 31–37. https://doi.org/10.3917/seve.054.0031

Clouston, S. A. P., & Link, B. G. (2021). A retrospective on fundamental cause theory: State of the literature and goals for the future. *Annual Review of Sociology, 47*(1), 131–156. https://doi.org/10.1146/annurev-soc-090320-094912

Crawford, R. (1994). The boundaries of the self and the unhealthy other: Relfections on health, culture and aids. *Social Science & Medicine, 38*(10), 1347–1365.

Crenshaw, K. (1989). Demarginalizing the intersection of race and sex: A black feminist critique of antidiscrimination doctrine, feminist theory and antiracist policies. *University of Chicago Legal Forum, 1989*(1), 139–167.

Cullati, S. (2014). The influence of work-family conflict trajectories on self-rated health trajectories in Switzerland: A life course approach. *Social Science & Medicine, 113*, 23–33. https://doi.org/10.1016/j.socscimed.2014.04.030

Cullati, S., Courvoisier, D. S., & Burton-Jeangros, C. (2014). Mental health trajectories and their embeddedness in work and family circumstances: A latent state-trait approach to life-course trajectories. *Sociology of Health & Illness, 36*(7), 1077–1094. https://doi.org/10.1111/1467-9566.12156

Curran, D. (2013). Risk society and the distribution of bads: Theorizing class in the risk society. *The British Journal of Sociology, 64*(1), 44–62. https://doi.org/10.1111/1468-4446.12004

Curran, D. (2018). Beck's creative challenge to class analysis: From the rejection of class to the discovery of risk-class. *Journal of Risk Research, 21*(1), 29–40. https://doi.org/10.1080/13669877.2017.1351464

Curran, D. (2022). *Handbook on risk and inequality*. Edward Elgar Publishing.

Davison, C., Frankel, S., & Davey Smith, G. (1992). The limits of lifestyle: Re-assessing « Fatalism » in the popular culture of illness prevention. *Social Science and Medicine, 34*(6), 675–685.

De Prez, V., Jolidon, V., Cullati, S., Burton-Jeangros, C., & Bracke, P. (2022). Cervical cancer (over-)screening in Europe: Balancing organised and opportunistic programmes. *Scandinavian Journal of Public Health, 51*, 1239–1247. https://doi.org/10.1177/14034948221118215

Di Fonzo, D., Fabri, A., & Pasetto, R. (2022). Distributive justice in environmental health hazards from industrial contamination: A systematic review of national and near-national assessments of social inequalities. *Social Science & Medicine, 297*, 114834. https://doi.org/10.1016/j.socscimed.2022.114834

Douglas, M. (1990). Risk as a forensic resource. *Daedalus, 119*(4), 1–16.

Dumas, A., Robitaille, J., & Jette, S. L. (2014). Lifestyle as a choice of necessity: Young women, health and obesity. *Social Theory & Health, 12*(2), 138–158. https://doi.org/10.1057/sth.2013.25

Duvoux, N., & Vezinat, N. (2023). Le concept de santé sociale: Une approche collective, méso-sociologique et intégrée du soin. *L'Année sociologique, 73*(2), 393–426. https://doi.org/10.3917/anso.232.0393

Ewald, F. (1986). *L'Etat providence.* Bernard Grasset.

Ferraro, K. F., & Shippee, T. P. (2009). Aging and cumulative inequality: How does inequality get under the skin? *The Gerontologist, 49*(3), 333–343. https://doi.org/10.1093/geront/gnp034

Finucane, M., Slovic, P., Mertz, C., Flynn, J., & Satterfield, T. (2000). Gender, race and perceived risk: The « white male effect ». *Health, Risk & Society, 2*(2), 159–172.

Fiske, A., Galasso, I., Eichinger, J., McLennan, S., Radhuber, I., Zimmermann, B., & Prainsack, B. (2022). The second pandemic: Examining structural inequality through reverberations of COVID-19 in Europe. *Social Science & Medicine, 292,* 114634. https://doi.org/10.1016/j.socscimed.2021.114634

Frohlich, K. L., & Potvin, L. (2008). Transcending the known in public health practice. *American Journal of Public Health, 98*(2), 216–221. https://doi.org/10.2105/AJPH.2007.114777

Giritli Nygren, K., & Olofsson, A. (2014). Intersectional approaches in health-risk research: A critical review. *Sociology Compass, 8*(9), 1112–1126. https://doi.org/10.1111/soc4.12176

Giritli Nygren, K., Olofsson, A., & Öhman, S. (2022). Actor, structure and inequality: An intersectional perspective of risk. In D. Curran (Ed.), *Handbook on risk and inequality*. Edward Elgar Publishing.

Gkiouleka, A., Huijts, T., Beckfield, J., & Bambra, C. (2018). Understanding the micro and macro politics of health: Inequalities, intersectionality & institutions - A research agenda. *Social Science & Medicine, 200*, 92–98. https://doi.org/10.1016/j.socscimed.2018.01.025

Grusky, D. (2019). The past, present and future of social inequalities. In *Social stratification, class, race, and gender in sociological perspective* (2nd ed., pp. 3–51). Routledge. https://doi.org/10.4324/9780429306419

Harris, K. M., & Schorpp, K. M. (2018). Integrating biomarkers in social stratification and health research. *Annual Review of Sociology, 44*(1), 361–386. https://doi.org/10.1146/annurev-soc-060116-053339

Herzlich, C. (1992). *Santé et maladie. Analyse d'une représentation sociale.* Editions de l'école des hautes études en sciences sociales.

Holman, D., & Walker, A. (2021). Understanding unequal ageing: Towards a synthesis of intersectionality and life course analyses. *European Journal of Ageing, 18*(2), 239–255. https://doi.org/10.1007/s10433-020-00582-7

Homan, P. (2019). Structural sexism and health in the United States: A new perspective on health inequality and the gender system. *American Sociological Review, 84*(3), 486–516. https://doi.org/10.1177/0003122419848723

Illich, I. (1975). *Némésis médicale. L'expropriation de la santé*. Seuil.

Jolidon, V., Bracke, P., & Burton-Jeangros, C. (2021). Macro-contextual determinants of cancer screening participation and inequalities: A multilevel analysis of 29 European countries. *SSM - Population Health, 15*, 100830. https://doi.org/10.1016/j.ssmph.2021.100830

Jouzel, J.-N., & Dedieu, F. (2013). Rendre visible et laisser dans l'ombre: Savoir et ignorance dans les politiques de santé au travail. *Revue française de science politique, 63*(1), 29–49. https://doi.org/10.3917/rfsp.631.0029

Kelly-Irving, M., & Delpierre, C. (2021). Framework for understanding health inequalities over the life course: The embodiment dynamic and biological mechanisms of exogenous and endogenous origin. *Journal of Epidemiology and Community Health, 75*(12), 1181–1186. https://doi.org/10.1136/jech-2021-216430

Krieger, N., Chen, J. T., Waterman, P. D., Hartman, C., Stoddard, A. M., Quinn, M. M., Sorensen, G., & Barbeau, E. M. (2008). The inverse hazard law: Blood pressure, sexual harassment, racial discrimination, workplace abuse and occupational exposures in US low-income black, white and Latino workers. *Social Science & Medicine, 67*(12), 1970–1981. https://doi.org/10.1016/j.socscimed.2008.09.039

Link, B. G., & Phelan, J. (1995). Social conditions as fundamental causes of disease. *Journal of Health and Social Behavior, 35*, 80. https://doi.org/10.2307/2626958

Machů, V., Arends, I., Veldman, K., & Bültmann, U. (2022). Work-family trajectories and health: A systematic review. *Advances in Life Course Research, 52*, 100466. https://doi.org/10.1016/j.alcr.2022.100466

Mann, J. M. (1997). Medicine and public health, ethics and human rights. *The Hastings Center Report, 27*(3), 6–13.

Marmot, M. (2004). *Status syndrome: How your social standing directly affects your health and life expectancy*. Bloomsbury.

Marmot, M., Friel, S., Bell, R., Houweling, T. A., & Taylor, S. (2008). Closing the gap in a generation: Health equity through action on the social determinants of health. *The Lancet, 372*(9650), 1661–1669. https://doi.org/10.1016/S0140-6736(08)61690-6

Marmot, M. G., & Wilkinson, R. G. (Eds.). (1999). *Social determinants of health*. Oxford University Press.

Mendenhall, E., Newfield, T., & Tsai, A. C. (2022). Syndemic theory, methods, and data. *Social Science & Medicine, 295*, 114656. https://doi.org/10.1016/j.socscimed.2021.114656

Mongin, D., Cullati, S., Kelly-Irving, M., Rosselet, M., Regard, S., & Courvoisier, D. S. (2022). Neighbourhood socio-economic vulnerability and access to COVID-19 healthcare during the first two waves of the pandemic in Geneva, Switzerland: A gender perspective. *eClinicalMedicine, 46*, 101352. https://doi.org/10.1016/j.eclinm.2022.101352

Morioka, R. (2014). Gender difference in the health risk perception of radiation from Fukushima in Japan: The role of hegemonic masculinity. *Social Science & Medicine, 107*, 105–112. https://doi.org/10.1016/j.socscimed.2014.02.014

Neufcourt, L., Castagné, R., Mabile, L., Khalatbari-Soltani, S., Delpierre, C., & Kelly-Irving, M. (2022). Assessing how social exposures are integrated in exposome research: A scoping review. *Environmental Health Perspectives, 130*(11), 116001. https://doi.org/10.1289/EHP11015

Olofsson, A., Zinn, J. O., Griffin, G., Nygren, K. G., Cebulla, A., & Hannah-Moffat, K. (2014). The mutual constitution of risk and inequalities: Intersectional risk theory. *Health, Risk & Society, 16*(5), 417–430. https://doi.org/10.1080/13698575.2014.942258

Petersen, A., & Lupton, D. (1996). *The new public health. Health and self in the age of risk*. Sage.

Pfefferkorn, R. (2007). *Inégalités et rapports sociaux. Rapports de classes, rapports de sexes*. La Dispute.

Piketty, T. (2017). *Capital in the twenty-first century* (A. Goldhammer, Trans.). The Belknap Press of Harvard University Press.

Ranci, C. (2010). *Social vulnerability in Europe: The new configuration of social risks*. Palgrave Macmillan. http://public.eblib.com/choice/publicfullrecord.aspx?p=578907

Rasborg, K. (2022). *Chapter 5: Changing risks, individualisation and inequality in a recast welfare state* (pp. 70–87). Edward Elgar Publishing. https://doi.org/10.4337/9781788972260.00013

Refle, J.-E., Fakhoury, J., Burton-Jeangros, C., Consoli, L., & Jackson, Y. (2023). Impact of legal status regularization on undocumented migrants' self-reported and mental health in Switzerland. *SSM - Population Health, 22*, 101398. https://doi.org/10.1016/j.ssmph.2023.101398

Riou, J., Panczak, R., Althaus, C. L., Junker, C., Perisa, D., Schneider, K., Criscuolo, N. G., Low, N., & Egger, M. (2021). Socioeconomic position and the COVID-19 care cascade from testing to mortality in Switzerland: A population-based analysis. *The Lancet Public Health, 6*(9), e683–e691. https://doi.org/10.1016/S2468-2667(21)00160-2

Savage, M., Dumas, A., & Stuart, S. A. (2013). Fatalism and short-termism as cultural barriers to cardiac rehabilitation among underprivileged men. *Sociology of Health & Illness, 35*(8), 1211–1226. https://doi.org/10.1111/1467-9566.12040

Shields, S. A. (2008). Gender: An intersectionality perspective. *Sex Roles, 59*, 301–311.

Sieber, S., Orsholits, D., Cheval, B., Ihle, A., Kelly-Irving, M., Delpierre, C., Burton-Jeangros, C., & Cullati, S. (2021). Social protection expenditure on health in later life in 20 European countries: Spending more to reduce health inequalities. *Social Science & Medicine, 292*, 114569. https://doi.org/10.1016/j.socscimed.2021.114569

Siegrist, M., & Árvai, J. (2020). Risk perception: Reflections on 40 years of research. *Risk Analysis, 40*(S1), 2191–2206. https://doi.org/10.1111/risa.13599

Singer, M. (2011). Down cancer alley: The lived experience of health and environmental suffering in Louisiana's chemical corridor. *Medical Anthropology Quarterly, 25*(2), 141–163. https://doi.org/10.1111/j.1548-1387.2011.01154.x

Singer, M., Bulled, N., Ostrach, B., & Mendenhall, E. (2017). Syndemics and the biosocial conception of health. *The Lancet, 389*(10072), 941–950. https://doi.org/10.1016/S0140-6736(17)30003-X

Singer, M., & Clair, S. (2003). Syndemics and public health: Reconceptualizing disease in bio-social context. *Medical Anthropology Quarterly, 17*(4), 423–441. https://doi.org/10.2307/3655345

Singer, M., & Rylko-Bauer, B. (2021). The syndemics and structural violence of the COVID pandemic: Anthropological insights on a crisis. *Open Anthropological Research, 1*(1), 7–32. https://doi.org/10.1515/opan-2020-0100

Swidler, A. (1986). Culture in action: Symbols and strategies. *American Sociological Review, 51*(2), 273–286. https://doi.org/10.2307/2095521

Umamaheswar, J., & Tan, C. (2020). "Dad, wash your hands": Gender, care work, and attitudes toward risk during the COVID-19 pandemic. *Socius, 6*, 1–14. https://doi.org/10.1177/2378023120964376

Vargas, N., Mora, G. C., & Gleeson, S. (2023). Race and ideology in a pandemic: White privilege and patterns of risk perception during COVID-19. *Social Problems, 70*(1), 219–237. https://doi.org/10.1093/socpro/spab037

Vermeulen, R., Schymanski, E. L., Barabási, A.-L., & Miller, G. W. (2020). The exposome and health: Where chemistry meets biology. *Science, 367*(6476), 392–396. https://doi.org/10.1126/science.aay3164

Weber, M. (1964 [1904]). *L'éthique protestante et l'esprit du capitalisme: Suivi d'autres essais*. Plon. [1905 original version in German *Die protestantische Ethik und der Geist des Kapitalismus*].

Willems, B., Cullati, S., Prez, V. D., Jolidon, V., Burton-Jeangros, C., & Bracke, P. (2020). Cancer screening participation and gender stratification in Europe. *Journal of Health and Social Behavior, 61*(3), 377–395. https://doi.org/10.1177/0022146520938708

Wynne, B. (1996). May the sheep safely graze? A reflexive view of the expert-lay knowledge divide. In S. Lash, B. Wynne, & B. Szerszynski (Eds.), *Risk, environment and modernity: Towards a new ecology* (pp. 44–83). Sage.

7

Conclusion: Health and Risk in Social Contexts

This book focused on the challenges people encounter when they navigate the uncertainty of modern life, formulated in terms of risk predictions related to their health. Through the lens of social experiences of risks, I have been interested in how they manage to handle health risks and uncertainty through the elaboration of symbolic meanings, combining risk evidence, experiential or embodied knowledge, emotional reactions, and moral judgments that together support their concrete actions. These experiences are shaped by interactions with other people and by the dense institutional context in which medicine and public health specialists handle health issues. In relation with my own research on these issues, I mobilized empirical findings with the intention to better characterize the lived reality of health risks. The regularities observed across risks and contexts were developed into five chapters tackling what I consider to be important dimensions of health risk experiences.

First, it was shown how formulations of formal risk knowledge striving to produce certainty through numbers encounter numerous challenges when applied in concrete social circumstances. These include the limited relevance of probabilities in making personal decisions, an overall poor statistical or risk numeracy across society, and the awareness that

C. Burton-Jeangros, *Experiences of Health Risks*, Critical Studies in Risk and Uncertainty, https://doi.org/10.1007/978-3-031-65377-3_7

knowledge is partial as a result of deliberate manipulation or incapacity to make sense of it, especially in times of crises. In addition to the extent to which social influences impact scientific knowledge, individual and collective reflexivity keeps stressing the shortcomings of the quantification of risks. These elements contribute to unsettle people's trust in abstract systems, and the COVID-19 pandemic has been particularly emblematic of the difficulties to govern with risk calculations.

Second, the ambition to control risk through individual and collective efforts generates elevated expectations that do not systematically materialize. Constant attention toward the future, with a focus on adverse events, contributes to the contemporary sense of individual and collective vulnerability. Emotions are omnipresent in dealings with possible future damage and shape a cultural climate focused on pending collective catastrophes or missed opportunities for personal better health. Indeed, people do not remain neutral toward all these predictions, and their emotions reveal their individual or professional engagements toward what matters to them. Acknowledging the multiple roles emotions play in prevention programs and social practices might help to make them more explicit parts of the picture, as an important dimension of handling danger in society.

Third, people endorse or reject advice in diverse ways, based on risk predictions, depending on how it resonates with their own values and past experiences. At the same time, despite sharp criticisms formulated by a minority, the enduring authority of science can be observed in the constant justifications people formulate to explain why they do not comply with prevention recommendations, according to a range of reasons that can be self-centered, in the case of vaccine hesitancy, or more collective, when demanding justice in exposure to environmental hazards. People's constant negotiations between expressing their autonomy while paying attention to social rules formulated by prevention specialists show the continuous dynamic taking place between their agency and social constraints.

Fourth, people are influenced by others through how these respond to long-standing or emerging health threats. Othering in times of crisis is obviously pervasive, playing central functions in making sense of danger. It is present across society, serving some personal needs for ontological security while having detrimental effects on the more vulnerable. Institutions and professionals are not immune to these mechanisms, and they contribute to the reproduction of divisions and tensions in society through their framing of risks. In health matters, moral judgments are omnipresent, they reinforce one's identity but at the cost of 'spoiling' the identities of others (Goffman, 1990 [1963]).

Fifth, the role of social structures in all the above considerations has been further elaborated, emphasizing how power dynamics in society constantly shape exposure to risks and the responses people are able or willing to formulate. Despite the assumption that risks, especially global and pervasive ones like the pandemic or environmental change, would be blind to people's contrasted conditions, persistent inequalities show that differences in health are not solely produced by individual variations in biology, genetics, or behaviors. They result from vastly contrasting living conditions, whose respective advantages and disadvantages are maintained by the institutions themselves.

What conclusions can be offered regarding risk scholarship? I showed how much risk is unsettling the continuity of social life, generating tensions across contrasted goals, creating conflicts and alliances, as well as dilemmas in the definition of strategies to avert future harm. I adopted an emic perspective on risk, that is, a view from within (Brown, 2021). Moving beyond the long debate about the ontological status of risk opposing realist to constructivist positions, what matters is that risk "has materialized consequences in people's everyday lives" (Giritli Nygren et al., 2022, p. 108). Furthermore, I emphasized how these consequences are shaped by power dynamics between health institutions and members of the public, as well as across social categories placed in more or less privileged positions in social hierarchies. Such dynamics are however not restricted to health risks and they shape experiences of risks more broadly.

In a modern context dominated by statistical, medical, and psychological perspectives, people who do not act according to recommendations are often belittled when labeled ignorant, emotional, biased, selfish, complacent, or supporters of conspiracy theories. Such recurring judgments formulated by moral entrepreneurs may serve to consolidate their own position, put forth as the only legitimate one. In those contexts, the media also act as important players. On the one hand, they reflect the multiple facets of official positions, mixing facts and emotions. On the other hand, they fuel controversies by amplifying dissenting views, whether framed within traditional media formats or formulated autonomously when people use social media to challenge institutions. Across these dynamics, multiple interpretations of risk and uncertainty are conveyed, supporting reflexivity but also generating confusion.

In that context, social sciences provide important insights to question the relevance of constant risk surveillance and they encourage a reflexive monitoring of official and lay responses in modern society (Giddens, 1990, 1991). Indeed, as stated by Kleinman (2010), it is necessary to assess the unintended consequences of social actions. Illustrations provided across the chapters of this book have shown the presence of some deleterious effects of interventions put in place to prevent health risks. In some instances, prevention generates anxiety or leads to the manipulation of others through deliberate amplification or minimization of hazards, alongside paternalist justifications. Controversies around risks, which could by definition emerge later on, challenge the capacity to easily assess the relevance of multiple and contradictory claims. Recurrent observations of stigmatization toward others not only reproduce social divisions but also add to the preexisting burden of those having less resources and power in society, contributing to social and health inequalities. This raises important concerns as to the role played by prevention efforts. While it is crucial to identify social categories that are more exposed to health risks in order to improve their chances for good health, such a strategy contributes to setting frontiers and entails risks of essentialization of segments of the population through processes of categorizations. This emphasizes the importance of paying attention to relations across categories, since systems of privileges and disadvantages do not exist in themselves but are shaped by these relations.

Overall, I want to stress the importance of considering health risk prevention as a system of interactions, with an invitation to consider the role of institutions and their representatives in the regulation of risks. Along Becker and Horowitz (1972) observations a while ago already, research still tends to focus on the recipients of institutional action, with limited attention given to the role of experts and organizations: "ordinarily, the agency will not see its own operation as one of the causes of the problem, and thus those operations will not be included in the area the researcher agrees to study; by implications, he agrees not to study them" (p. 63). Nevertheless, the chapters in this book showed the relevance of considering how people tackle risks in both their professional or social roles, to which various forms of resources and advantages are attached. The regulation of health risks occurs amidst relations encompassing power dynamics that need to be unpacked. This stresses the importance of considering the role played by 'unmarked categories', as they are central to the way power and privileges are organized (Giritli Nygren et al., 2022). In that respect, qualitative studies are particularly important to document what happens in interactions, when social positions are constantly re-enacted through undermining moral judgments formulated toward others.

In times of crisis or in the face of unresolved issues, often associated with a lack of compliance with public health recommendations, health institutions seek help from the social sciences, but most of the time without questioning their own framing of the issue. Taking the contribution of the social sciences seriously however implies valuing the way they reformulate the problems to be addressed and accepting their theoretical and methodological frameworks. Participatory research, engaging concerned communities, in studies and in the elaboration of risk prevention offers other important avenues for a better tackling of health risks. These strategies are gaining more support across domains and can help to address the challenges of risk prevention. However, they challenge existing power dynamics and thus are not welcomed by all experts.

As a final point, what conclusions can be offered regarding the value of health in society? The increasing attention dedicated to risks means that being in good health is becoming increasingly elusive. The extension of formal risk knowledge over the past decades has clearly redefined the boundary between health and illness. Being healthy or being sick used to be thought of as two distinct states, distinguished by the respective absence or presence of symptoms or tangible signs of a nonoptimal state. Leriche's (1936) statement of health as "life in the silence of the organs" (in Canguilhem, 1999 [1943], p. 52) well illustrates such an embodied or sensory dimension of health. In contrast, the advent of 'at-risk' status places health and disease on a continuum entailing a range of intermediate states where individuals are no longer "ill" but are not completely "healthy" either. In those intermediate states, people are increasingly dependent on specialists and technical devices (genetic sequencing, statistical analysis) to establish their health status. This extension contributes to unsettling the experience of health, and it has become common today that people question their own feelings of good health, thinking that if they were put under systematic medical investigation, they would probably be diagnosed with one or more conditions that are currently silent.

Risk introduces the idea of something potentially wrong that one should be attentive to beyond her or his own perceptions. This reduces the trust one can have in how she or he is feeling since knowledge about the self is increasingly mediated through others, health specialists, the media, or technical devices. This was expressed by this HIV-infected woman who is told by doctors that she is healthy since her viremia (presence of HIV in blood) is undetectable while she experiences symptoms. She thus reflected: 'What is the basis for saying that you're "healthy"? Medical tests or how do I feel?' (Fargnoli, 2021, p. 196). Such an absence of trust in one's own body could contribute to explain the larger movement of declining trust toward institutions and others in general, as it is observed today.

Hence, probabilities or numbers provided in test results dissolve the experience of health: it becomes a vicarious or mediated experience depending on a range of technologies, and the body experiences are devalued. This can be related to the common observation that when one goes to a doctor, machines and tests have replaced physical examination and dialog. Caduff (2014) discusses the emphasis on 'biological vulnerability' associated with re-emerging infectious diseases and the biosecurity agenda. I believe, however, that this idea more broadly covers all domains of health. Debates about risk management around technological vulnerability flourished in the 1970s. In that context, Douglas and Wildawsky (1983) stated, "In the amazingly short space of fifteen to twenty years, confidence about the physical world has turned into doubt" (p. 10). This trend can now be applied to health and the individual body. Biological vulnerability invites each one of us to be alert and act appropriately in everyday life in compliance with recommendations based on the most recent evidence established on a number of people, instead of trusting one's own perceptions. Biological vulnerability encompasses a large range of conditions, from the early detection of the progressive onset of non-communicable diseases (such as cancer), inscribed in the individual body, possibly including its genetic make-up, to being ready for sudden global health events (such as the COVID-19 pandemic) impacting all of society. Risk knowledge constantly produces and refines projections of possible disorders, fueled by further developments in expertise and technologies. It thus promotes a relation to health that is very remote from the positive definition of the World Health Organization constitution in 1946, considering health as "a state of complete physical, mental and social well-being and not merely the absence of disease or infirmity". As stated in the introduction of the book, risk probabilities by definition take some distance from the actual experience of people, as regard their health but more broadly.

Indeed, the focus on health as an individual enterprise, achieved through personal efforts, reflects the climate of individualization and is well aligned with the powerful medical perspective which approaches individual bodies as detached from their social environment. However, beyond its individual importance, health is a major collective resource for society. Health inequalities reveal the tight interactions that exist between societal conditions of living and health. Hence, health issues largely overtake the expertise of medicine and concern society at large. This justifies the constant efforts of public health to mitigate diverse risks through strategies that rest on solidarity across segments of society, hence possibly redistributing resources and questioning the value of autonomy. Overall, the promotion of population health is a major societal goal requiring collective engagements and alliances. The social sciences question taken-for-granted or unchallenged prevention interventions, inviting us to pay attention to their individual and collective sometimes counterproductive consequences. They also unveil the changing power relations between institutions and individuals, in a complex dynamic fueled by difficulties and fears with regard to the actual capacity to control adverse future events. I hope that this book has convincingly shown that the social sciences have important contributions to offer in the policy thinking about health and risk governance.

References

Becker, H. S., & Horowitz, I. L. (1972). Radical politics and sociological research: Observations on methodology and ideology. *American Journal of Sociology, 78*(1), 48–66.

Brown, P. (2021). *On vulnerability: A critical introduction* (1st ed.). Routeldge.

Caduff, C. (2014). On the verge of death: Visions of biological vulnerability*. *Annual Review of Anthropology, 43*(1), 105–121. https://doi.org/10.1146/annurev-anthro-102313-030341

Canguilhem, G. (1999). *Le normal et le pathologique*. Presses universitaires de France.

Douglas, M., & Wildawsky, A. (1983). *Risk and culture: An essay on the selection of technological and environmental dangers*. University of California Press.

Fargnoli, V. (2021). *InVIHsibles: Trajectoires de femmes séropositives*. Editions Antipodes.

Giddens, A. (1990). *The consequences of modernity*. Polity Press.

Giddens, A. (1991). *Modernity and self-identity in the late modern age*. Polity Press.

Giritli Nygren, K., Olofsson, A., & Öhman, S. (2022). Actor, structure and inequality: An intersectional perspective of risk. In D. Curran (Ed.), *Handbook on risk and inequality*. Edward Elgar Publishing.

Goffman, E. (1990). *Stigma: Notes on the management of spoiled identity*. Penguin.

Kleinman, A. (2010). Four social theories for global health. *The Lancet, 375*(9725), 1518–1519. https://doi.org/10.1016/S0140-6736(10)60646-0

Index

C. Burton-Jeangros, *Experiences of Health Risks*, Critical Studies in Risk and Uncertainty, https://doi.org/10.1007/978-3-031-65377-3